MW01405442

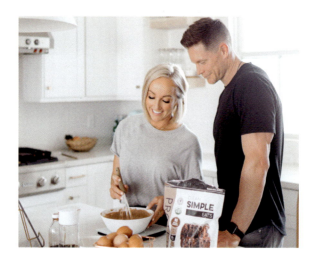

We have been hard at work behind the scenes to create this Summer Edition Clean Simple Treats book and we could not be more excited to share it with you! This book is filled with all of our summer favorites. We've included everything from simple cookies, bars and party treats you can whip up with your kids, to cakes, pies and cobblers that you can share with a crowd. We even added in all of our healthy, macro-balanced shake recipes and low-calorie refreshers for you to enjoy daily. We hope that your family falls in love with these healthier treat recipes like we have!

Enjoy! XO Erika & JJ

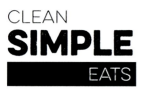

STAY CONNECTED

 @cleansimpleeats

 facebook.com/groups/cleansimpleeats

 hello@cleansimpleeats.com

 www.cleansimpleeats.com

For a list of cookie scoops we use, pans we love, and where to purchase some of the harder to find ingredients found in this book, visit our website: cleansimpleeats.com/products-we-love.

RECIPE

INDEX

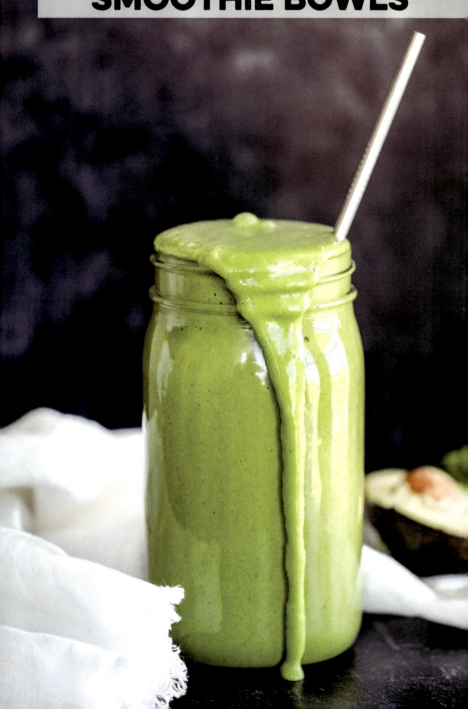

SHAKES & SMOOTHIE BOWLS

DRINK RESPONSIBLY

DON'T SPILL YOUR PROTEIN SHAKE!

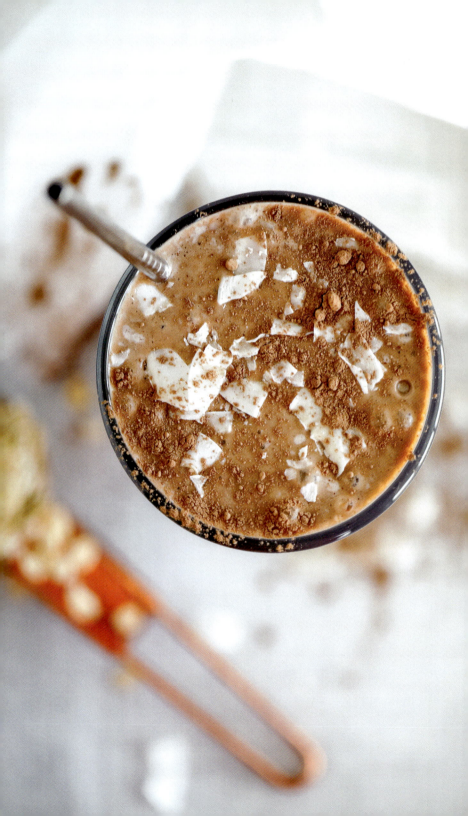

ALMOND JOY PROTEIN SHAKE

Makes 1 serving
345 calories / 11.5F / 34.5C / 25.5P

1 cup unsweetened almond milk
1 serving CSE Brownie Batter Protein Powder
2 Tbs. old-fashioned rolled oats
60g frozen banana slices
1 Tbs. cocoa powder
1 Tbs. unsweetened shredded coconut
½ Tbs. OffBeat Midnight Almond Coconut Butter
   or natural almond butter
½ tsp. vanilla extract
½ tsp. coconut extract
6-8 (120g) ice cubes

1. Add all of the ingredients to a high-powered blender. Blend on high until smooth.

2. Pour into a cup and enjoy!

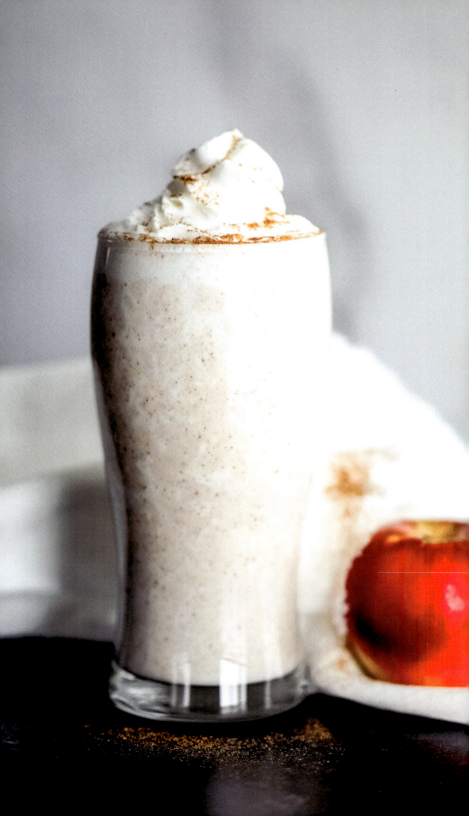

APPLE CRISP SMOOTHIE

Makes 1 serving
240 calories / 8F / 26C / 16P

¾ cup unsweetened almond milk
75g fresh, chopped apples
¼ cup fat-free cottage cheese
2 Tbs. old-fashioned rolled oats
2 Tbs. (8g) CSE Simply Vanilla Protein Powder
½ Tbs. OffBeat Cinnamon Bun Butter
   or natural almond butter
½ tsp. butter extract
½ tsp. cinnamon
8-10 (130g) ice cubes
Topping:
2 Tbs. spray whipped cream

1. Add all of the ingredients to a high-powered blender. Blend on high until smooth.

2. Pour into a cup, top with whipped cream and enjoy!

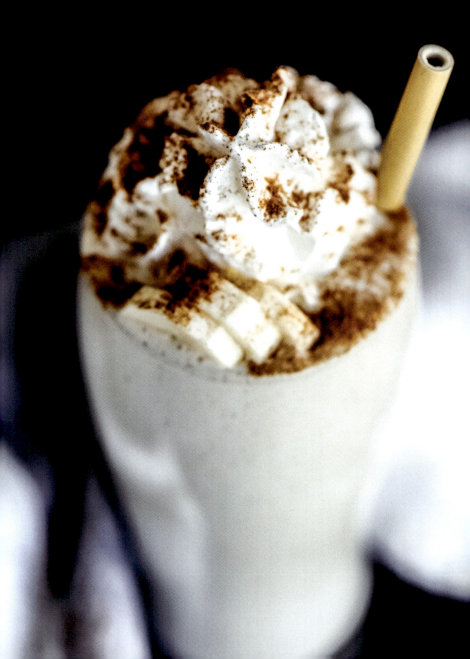

BANANAS FOSTER MILKSHAKE

Makes 1 serving
350 calories / 12F / 34C / 28P

---

1 cup unsweetened almond milk
1 serving CSE Bananas Foster or Simply Vanilla Protein Powder
75g frozen banana slices
2 Tbs. low-fat cottage cheese
2 Tbs. old-fashioned rolled oats
1 Tbs. OffBeat Cinnamon Bun Butter
   or natural almond butter
8-10 (120g) ice cubes
Topping:
2 Tbs. spray whipped cream
Dash cinnamon

1. Add all of the ingredients to a high-powered blender. Blend on high until smooth.

2. Pour into a cup. Top with whipped cream and a dash of cinnamon. Enjoy!

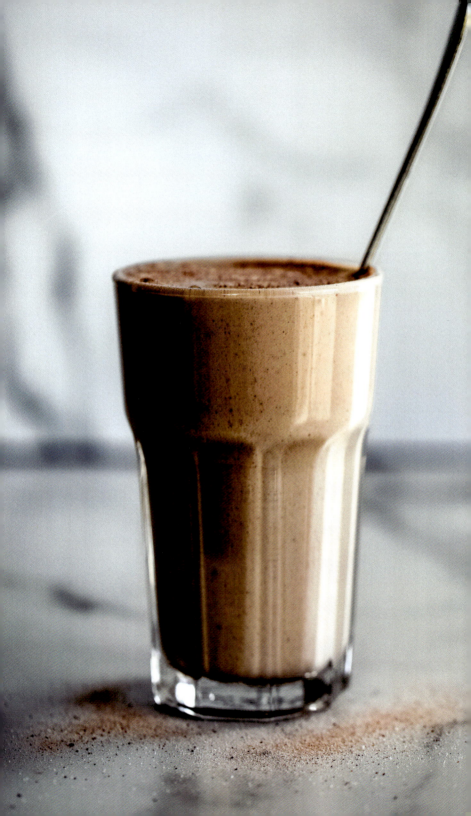

BERRY CHOCOLATEY SHAKE (POST-WORKOUT)

Makes 1 serving
216 calories / 0F / 27C / 28P

---

1 cup fat-free milk
1 ½ servings CSE Brownie Batter
   or Chocolate Peanut Butter Protein Powder
1 serving CSE Super Berry Mix
¼ tsp. xanthan gum
6-8 (120g) ice cubes

1. Add all of the ingredients to a high-powered blender. Blend on high until smooth.

2. Pour into a cup and enjoy right after a workout.

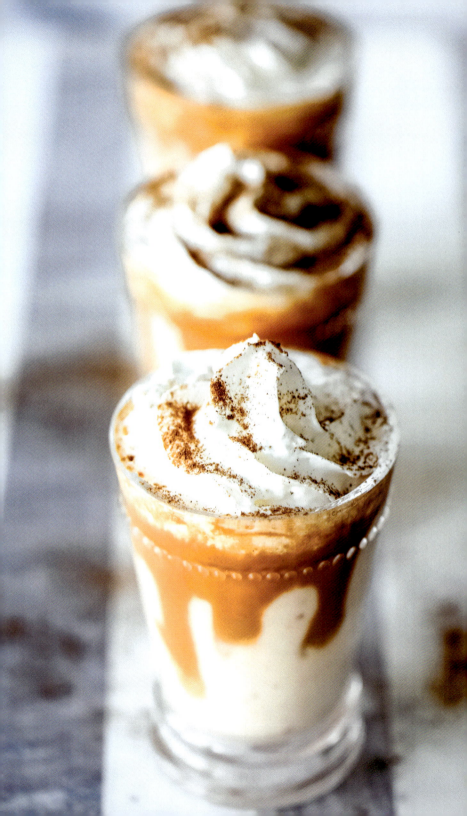

CARAMEL APPLE MILKSHAKE

Makes 1 serving
230 calories / 9F / 24C / 16P

½ cup unsweetened almond milk
½ cup low-fat cottage cheese
100g fresh, chopped apples
½ Tbs. OffBeat Salted Caramel Butter
   or natural almond butter
1 Tbs. CSE Caramel Toffee Protein Powder
   or sugar-free butterscotch pudding mix
Dash cinnamon
Vanilla stevia drops, to taste
12 (140g) ice cubes

Topping:
2 Tbs. spray whipped cream
Walden Farms Caramel Syrup, optional

1. Add all of the ingredients to a high-powered blender. Blend on high until smooth.

2. Pour into a cup, top with whipped cream and caramel syrup. Enjoy!

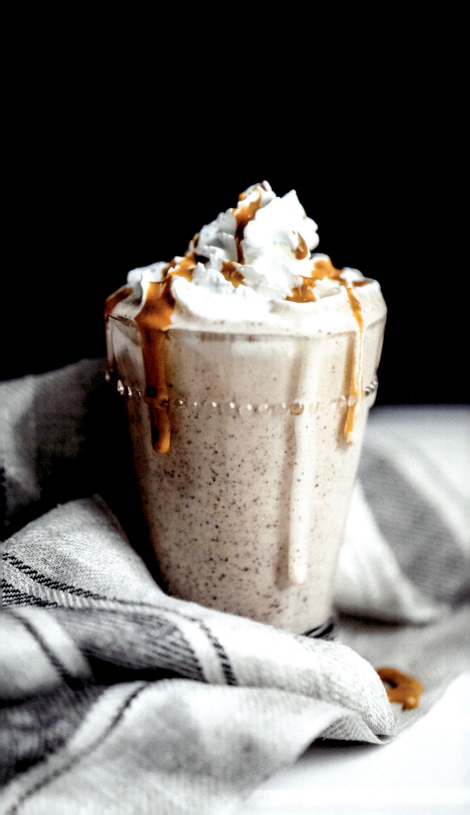

CARAMEL MOCHA MILKSHAKE

Makes 1 serving
250 calories / 9F / 23C / 21.5P

½ cup fat-free milk
1 Tbs. Crio Bru grounds, optional
1 Tbs. OffBeat Almond Mocha Butter, Salted Caramel Butter,
   Caramel Pecan Cluster Butter, or natural almond butter
½ serving (17g) CSE Brownie Batter
   or Caramel Toffee Protein Powder
¼ cup Sea Salt Caramel Halo Top ice cream
6-8 (120g) ice cubes
Topping:
2 Tbs. spray whipped cream

1. Add all of the ingredients to a high-powered blender. Blend on high until smooth.

2. Pour into a cup and top with spray whipped cream.

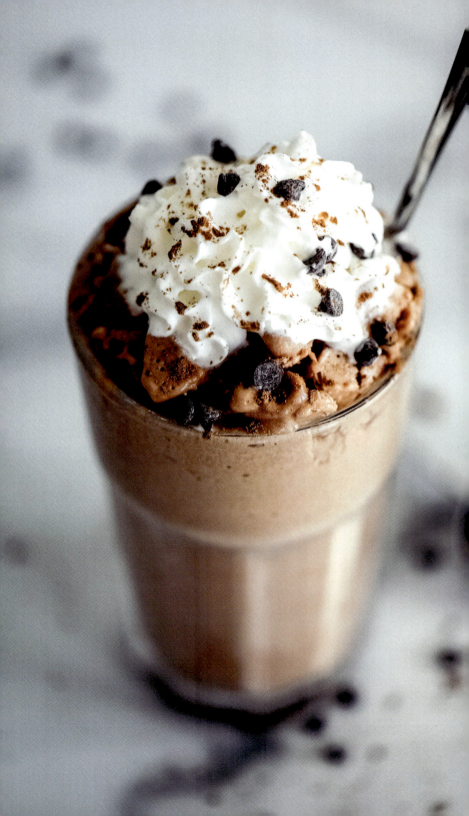

CHOCOLATE CARAMEL TOFFEE MILKSHAKE

Makes 1 serving
230 calories / 7F / 19C / 22P

1 cup vanilla almond milk
1 serving CSE Caramel Toffee Protein Powder
1 Tbs. cocoa powder
¼ tsp. xanthan gum
8-10 (160g) ice cubes
Topping:
2 Tbs. spray whipped cream
2 tsp. mini chocolate chips

1. Add all of the ingredients to a high-powered blender. Blend on high until smooth.

2. Pour into a cup and top with spray whipped cream and chocolate chips. It should be thick and creamy. Enjoy with a spoon!

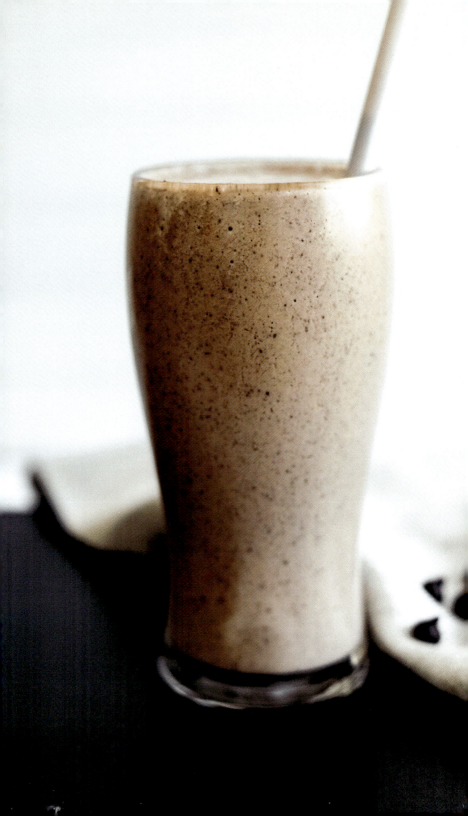

CHOCOLATE CHIP ALMOND MOCHA SHAKE

Makes 1 serving
350 calories / 12F / 33C / 27P

½ cup unsweetened almond milk
½ cup cold brewed coffee or cold brewed Crio Bru
¾ serving (24g) CSE Brownie Batter Protein Powder
100g frozen banana slices
2 Tbs. nonfat, plain Greek yogurt
1 Tbs. OffBeat Almond Mocha Butter
   or natural almond butter
15 extra dark chocolate chips
¼ tsp. almond extract, optional
6-8 (120g) ice cubes

1. Add all of the ingredients to a high-powered blender. Blend on high until smooth.

2. Pour into a cup and enjoy!

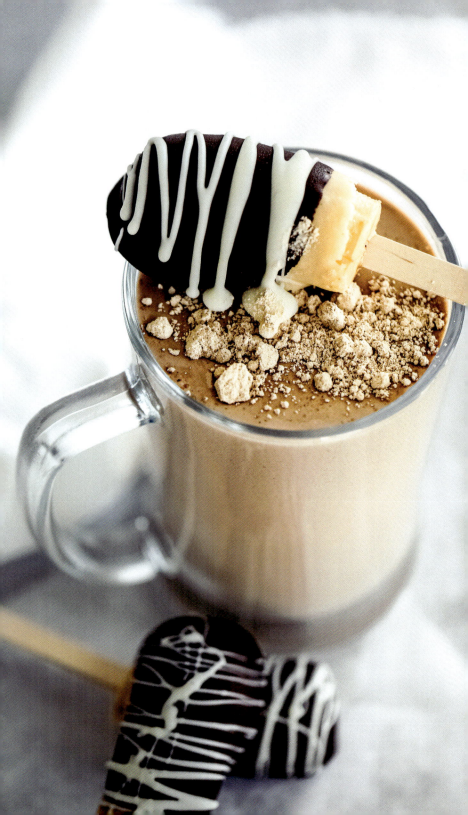

CHOCOLATE COVERED BANANA SHAKE

Makes 1 serving
220 calories / 4F / 20C / 27P

1 cup chocolate almond milk
1 serving CSE Bananas Foster Protein Powder
2 Tbs. chocolate peanut butter powder
30g frozen bananas
8-10 (130g) ice cubes

1. Add all of the ingredients to a blender. Blend on high until smooth.

2. Pour into a cup and enjoy!

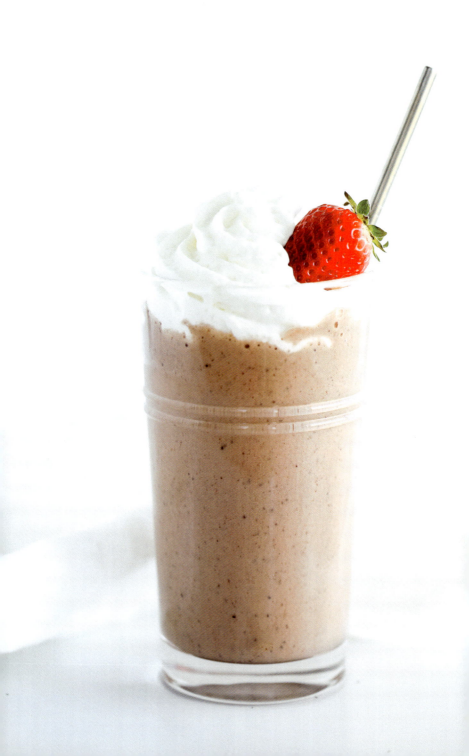

CHOCOLATE COVERED BERRY SHAKE
Makes 1 serving
216 calories / 4.5F / 21C / 22.5P

½ cup water
1 serving (34g) CSE Brownie Batter
   or Strawberry Cheesecake Protein Powder
1 Tbs. (16g) OffBeat Midnight Almond Coconut Butter
   Buckeye Brownie Peanut Butter, or dark chocolate chips
1 serving (10g) CSE Super Berry Mix
¼ tsp. xanthan gum, optional for thickness
6-8 (120g) ice cubes
Topping:
2 Tbs. spray whipped cream

1. Add all of the ingredients to a high-powered blender. Blend on high until smooth.

2. Pour into a cup, top with whipped cream and enjoy!

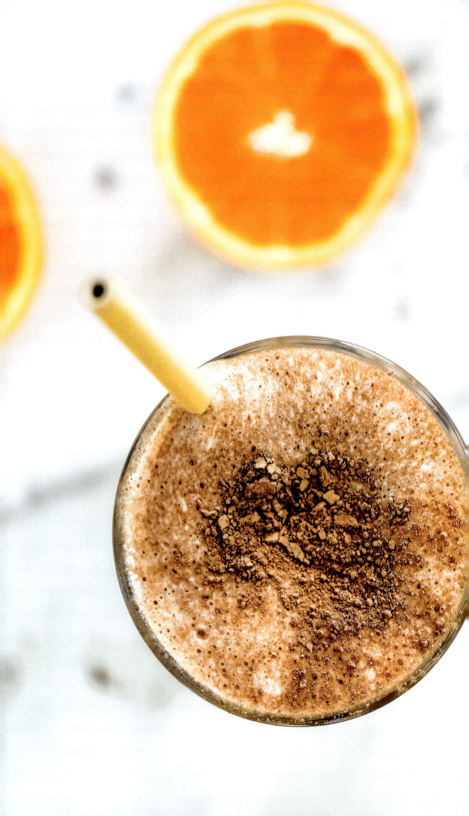

CHOCOLATE COVERED ORANGE SHAKE
(POST-WORKOUT)
Makes 1 serving
233 calories / 2F / 28C / 26P

¾ cup unsweetened almond milk
¼ cup fresh orange juice
1 clementine orange
1 serving CSE Brownie Batter Protein Powder
1 serving CSE Peach Mango Super Collagen Mix
½ Tbs. cocoa powder
Dash of xanthan gum, optional for added thickness
6-8 (120g) ice cubes

1. Add all of the ingredients to a high-powered blender. Blend on high until smooth.

2. Pour into a cup and enjoy after a workout!

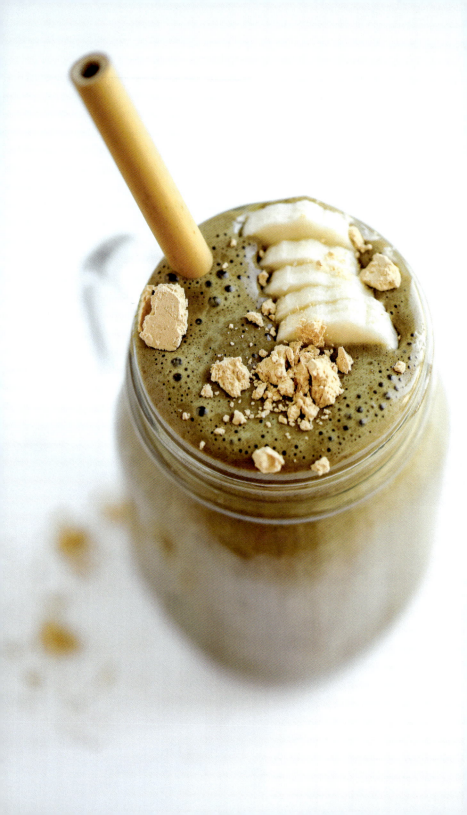

CHOCOLATE PEANUT BUTTER SHAKE

Makes 1 serving
245 calories / 7F / 25C / 20P

---

1 cup unsweetened cashew milk
½ serving (17g) CSE Brownie Batter
    or Chocolate Peanut Butter Protein Powder
½ Tbs. OffBeat Sweet Classic Peanut Butter
    or natural peanut butter
2 Tbs. powdered peanut butter
50g frozen banana slices
1 Tbs. cocoa powder
1 cup spinach
6-8 (120g) ice cubes

1. Add all of the ingredients to a high-powered blender. Blend on high until smooth.

2. Pour into a cup and enjoy!

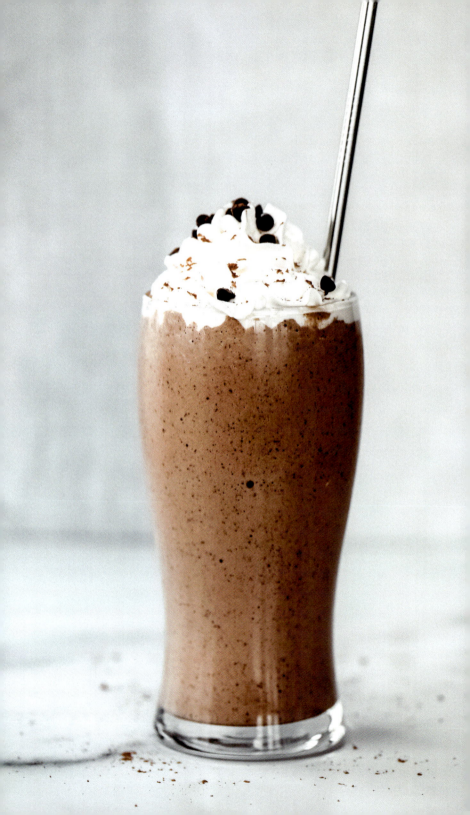

CHOCOLATE SPECKLED FROSTY

Makes 1 serving
240 calories / 7F / 25C / 18.5P

⅔ cup unsweetened almond milk
½ serving (16g) CSE Brownie Batter Protein Powder
50g frozen banana slices
¼ cup low-fat cottage cheese
10g dark chocolate chips
1 tsp. cocoa powder
½ tsp. vanilla extract
10-12 (150g) ice cubes
Topping:
2 Tbs. spray whipped cream

1. Add all of the ingredients to a high-powered blender. Blend on high until smooth.

2. Pour into a cup, top with whipped cream and enjoy!

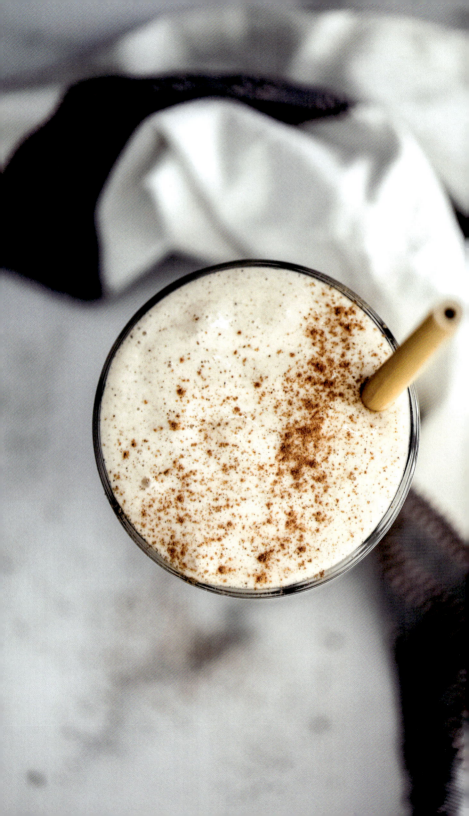

CINNAMON ROLL SHAKE

Makes 1 serving
350 calories / 12F / 34.5C / 26.5P

¾ cup unsweetened almond milk
¼ cup nonfat, plain Greek yogurt
¾ serving CSE Simply Vanilla or Cinnamon Roll Protein Powder
50g frozen banana slices
2 Tbs. old-fashioned rolled oats
1 Tbs. OffBeat Cinnamon Bun Butter
  or 3 Tbs. Neufchâtel cream cheese
1 tsp. coconut sugar
1 tsp. cinnamon
6-8 (120g) ice cubes

1. Add all of the ingredients to a high-powered blender. Blend on high until smooth.

2. Pour into a cup and enjoy!

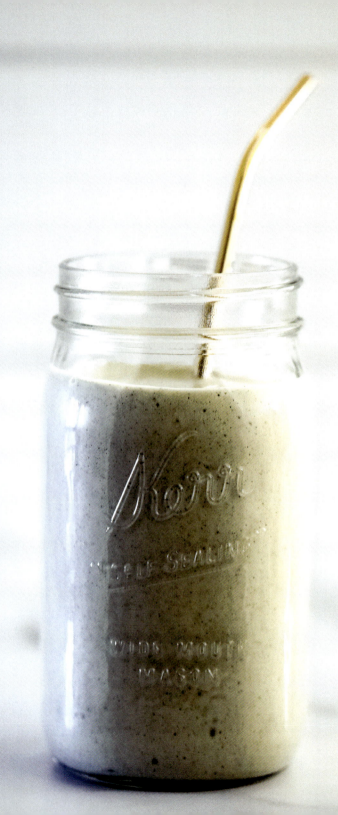

CREAMY GREENS BERRY SHAKE
(POST-WORKOUT)
Makes 1 serving
200 calories / 2.5F / 22C / 25P

---

1 cup unsweetened almond milk
2 Tbs. low-fat cottage cheese
1 serving CSE Simply Vanilla
   or Strawberry Cheesecake Protein Powder
1 serving CSE Super Greens Mix
1 serving CSE Super Berry Mix
Vanilla stevia drops, to taste
Dash of xanthan gum, to thicken
6-8 (120g) ice cubes

1. Add all of the ingredients to a high-powered blender. Blend on high until smooth.

2. Pour into a cup and enjoy after a workout!

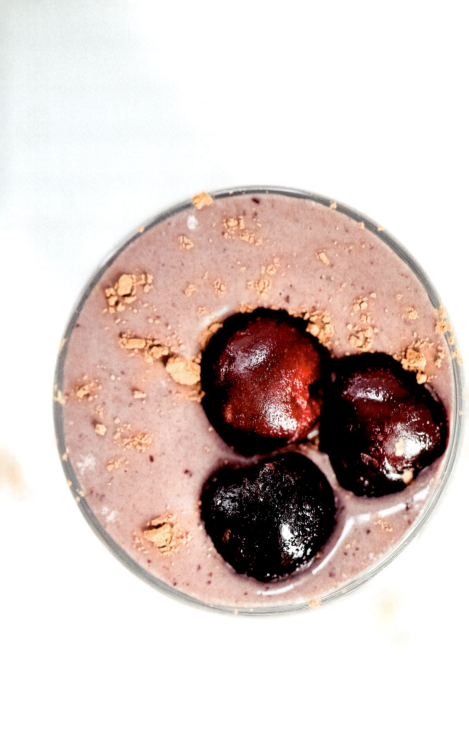

DARK CHOCOLATE CHERRY SHAKE

Makes 1 serving
245 calories / 8F / 23C / 20P

1 cup unsweetened almond milk
½ cup (70g) frozen, pitted, dark sweet cherries
¾ serving (24g) CSE Brownie Batter Protein Powder
1 Tbs. cocoa powder
½ Tbs. OffBeat Almond Mocha Butter,
    Midnight Almond Coconut Butter,
    or natural almond butter
6-8 (120g) ice cubes

1. Add all of the ingredients to a high-powered blender. Blend on high until smooth.

2. Pour into a cup and enjoy!

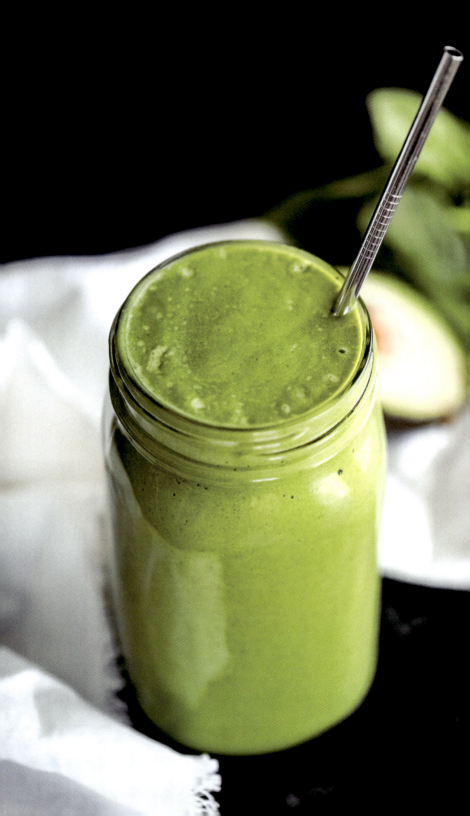

HULK POWER SHAKE

Makes 1 serving
350 calories / 13F / 34C / 25P

---

1 cup unsweetened almond milk
1 serving CSE Simply Vanilla Protein Powder
80g frozen banana slices
15g avocado
1 Tbs. OffBeat Butter of choice
    or natural almond butter
1 cup spinach
1 tsp. cinnamon
6-8 (120g) ice cubes

1. Add all of the ingredients to a high-powered blender. Blend on high until smooth.

2. Pour into a cup and enjoy!

*Add 1 serving of the CSE Super Greens Mix for an immunity boost or to increase your daily veggie intake!

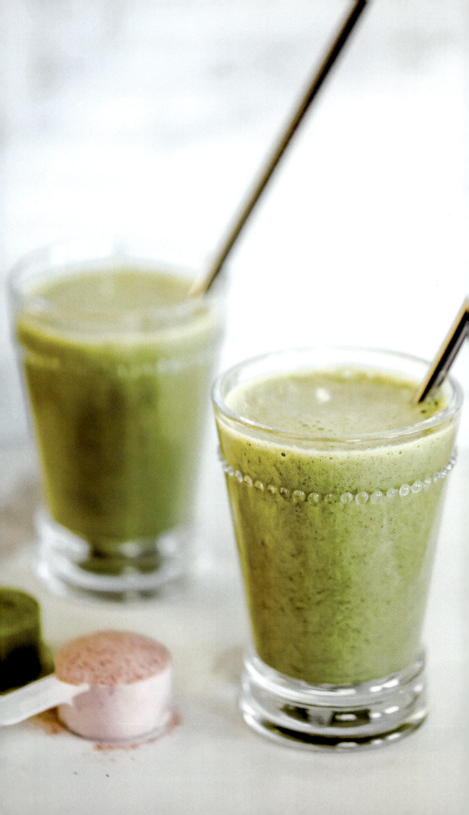

IMMUNITY BOOST SHAKE (POST-WORKOUT)

Makes 1 serving
223 calories / 0F / 29.5C / 27P

½ cup fat-free milk
¼ cup fresh orange juice
1 serving CSE Simply Vanilla Protein Powder
1 serving CSE Super Greens Mix
1 serving CSE Super Berry Mix
Vanilla stevia drops, to taste
Dash of xanthan gum, to thicken
6-8 (120g) ice cubes

1. Add all of the ingredients to a high-powered blender. Blend on high until smooth.

2. Pour into a cup and enjoy after a workout!

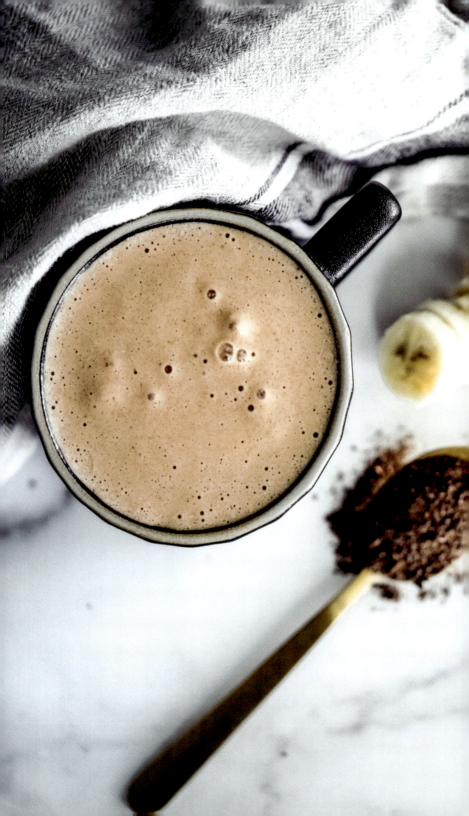

JAVA BANANA SHAKE

Makes 1 serving
250 calories / 8F / 26C / 18.5P

½ cup unsweetened almond milk
½ cup brewed Crio Bru or cold brewed black coffee
70g frozen banana slices
¾ serving (24g) CSE Brownie Batter Protein Powder
2 tsp. OffBeat Almond Mocha Butter,
    Midnight Almond Coconut Butter, or natural almond butter
6-8 (120g) ice cubes

1. Add all of the ingredients to a high-powered blender. Blend on high until smooth.

2. Pour into a cup and enjoy!

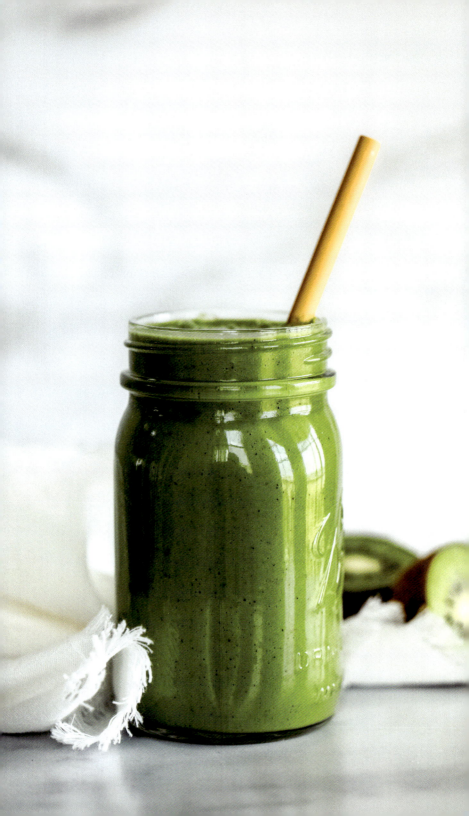

KIWI GREEN SMOOTHIE

Makes 1 serving
217 calories / 6F / 36C / 6.5P

½ cup plain kefir
¼ cup fresh orange juice
¼ cup cold water
1 serving CSE Super Greens Mix
1 cup baby spinach
50g pineapple
50g kiwi
30g avocado
½ lime, juice of
Vanilla stevia drops, to taste
8-10 (140g) ice cubes

1. Add all of the ingredients to a high-powered blender. Blend on high until smooth.

2. Pour into a cup and enjoy!

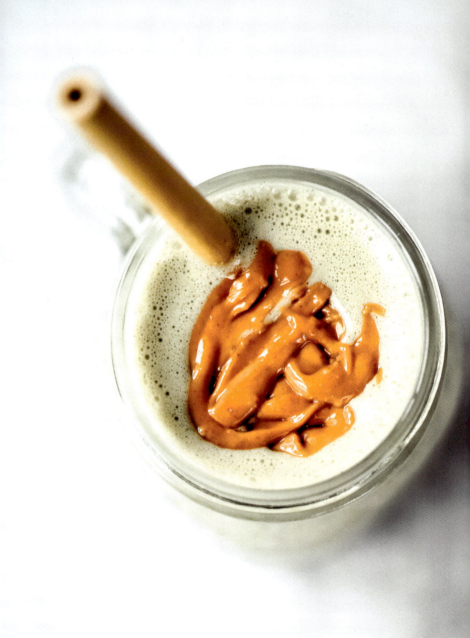

LEAN GREEN MUSCLE SHAKE

Makes 1 serving
227 calories / 7F / 25C / 17P

1 cup unsweetened almond milk
60g frozen banana slices
½ Tbs. OffBeat Sweet Classic Peanut Butter
  or natural peanut butter
½ serving (16g) CSE Protein Powder, any flavor
1 serving (9g) CSE Super Greens Mix
6-8 (120g) ice cubes

1. Add all of the ingredients to a high-powered blender. Blend on high until smooth.

2. Pour into a cup and enjoy!

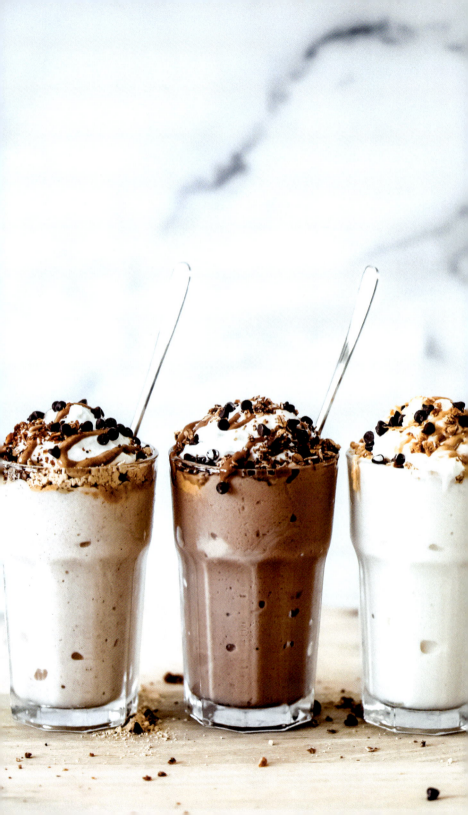

CHOCOLATE CARAMEL MIX-IN MILKSHAKE
Makes 1 serving
375 calories / 16F / 33C / 26P

Base:
1 cup unsweetened cashew milk
1 serving CSE Brownie Batter Protein Powder
1 Tbs. cocoa powder
¼ tsp. xanthan gum
150-160g ice cubes

Mix-ins:
25g Purely Elizabeth Maple + Almond Butter
   or Chocolate Sea Salt granola
10g OffBeat Salted Caramel Butter
   or natural almond butter
10g spray whipped cream
5g Enjoy Life mini chocolate chips

CHUNKY MONKEY MIX-IN MILKSHAKE
Makes 1 serving
400 calories / 16F / 35C / 28P

Base:
1 cup unsweetened cashew milk
1 serving CSE Bananas Foster Protein Powder
  or CSE Simply Vanilla Protein Powder
¼ tsp. xanthan gum
150-160g ice cubes

Mix-ins:
25g Purely Elizabeth Chocolate Sea Salt + Peanut Butter
   or Banana Nut granola
12g powdered peanut butter
10g OffBeat Sweet Classic Peanut Butter
   or natural peanut butter
10g spray whipped cream
5g Enjoy Life mini chocolate chips

1. Add all of the base ingredients to a high-powered blender. Blend on high until smooth.

2. Pour into a cup, top with mix-ins and enjoy with a spoon!

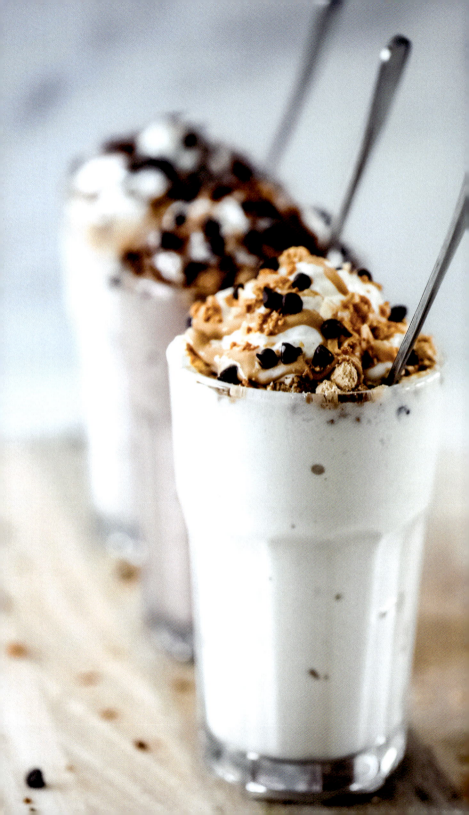

CINNAMON VANILLA MIX-IN MILKSHAKE
Makes 1 serving
355 calories / 15F / 32.5C / 25P

Base:
1 cup unsweetened cashew milk
1 serving CSE Simply Vanilla Protein Powder
¼ tsp. xanthan gum
150-160g ice cubes
Mix-ins:
25g Purely Elizabeth Original
   or Pumpkin Cinnamon granola
10g OffBeat Cinnamon Bun Butter
   or natural almond butter
10g spray whipped cream
5g Enjoy Life mini chocolate chips

DARK CHOCOLATE COCONUT MIX-IN MILKSHAKE
Makes 1 serving
410 calories / 18.5F / 34.5C / 26.5P

Base:
1 cup unsweetened cashew milk
1 serving CSE Brownie Batter Protein Powder
1 Tbs. cocoa powder
¼ tsp. xanthan gum
150-160g ice cubes
Mix-ins:
25g Purely Elizabeth Coconut Cashew
  or Chocolate Sea Salt granola
10g OffBeat Midnight Almond Coconut Butter
   or natural coconut butter
10g spray whipped cream
5g unsweetened flaked coconut
5g Enjoy Life mini chocolate chips

1. Add all of the base ingredients to a high-powered blender. Blend on high until smooth.

2. Pour into a cup, top with mix-ins and enjoy with a spoon!

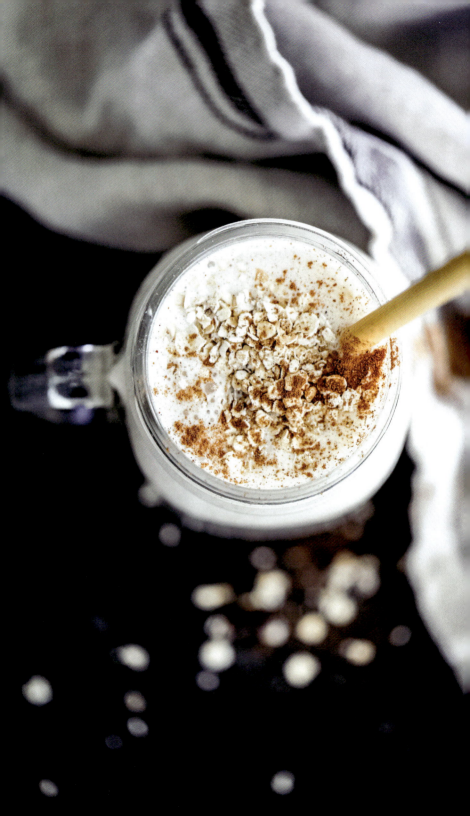

OATMEAL COOKIE SHAKE

Makes 1 serving
350 calories / 12F / 35.5C / 26P

---

1 cup unsweetened almond milk
½ serving CSE Simply Vanilla Protein Powder
⅓ cup old-fashioned rolled oats
⅓ cup low-fat cottage cheese
10g raisins
2 tsp. OffBeat Cinnamon Bun Butter,
    Gingerbread Cookie Butter or natural almond butter
1 tsp. cinnamon
Dash sea salt
⅛ tsp. butter extract
6-8 (120g) ice cubes

1. Add all of the ingredients to a high-powered blender. Blend on high until smooth.

2. Pour into a cup and enjoy!

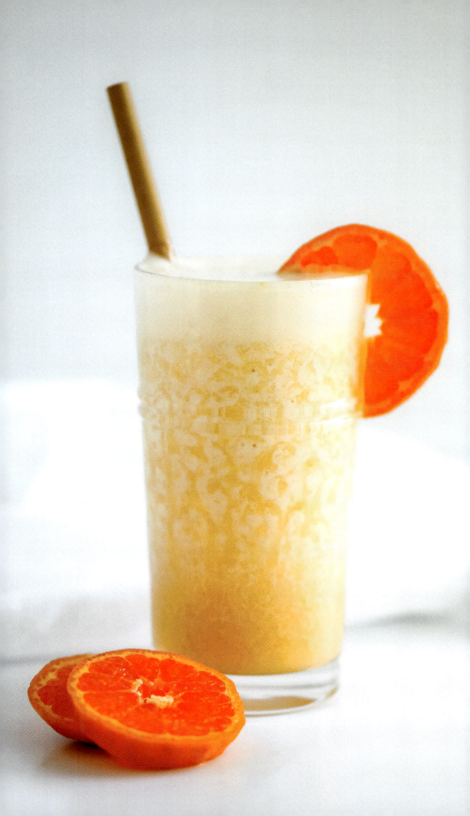

ORANGE JULIUS
(POST-WORKOUT)
Makes 1 serving
233 calories / 1.5F / 33C / 27P

½ cup unsweetened cashew milk
½ cup fresh orange juice
1 serving CSE Simply Vanilla Protein Powder
1 serving CSE Peach Mango Super Collagen Mix
30g frozen bananas
6-8 (120g) ice cubes

1. Add all of the ingredients to a high-powered blender. Blend on high until smooth.

2. Pour into a cup and enjoy after a workout!

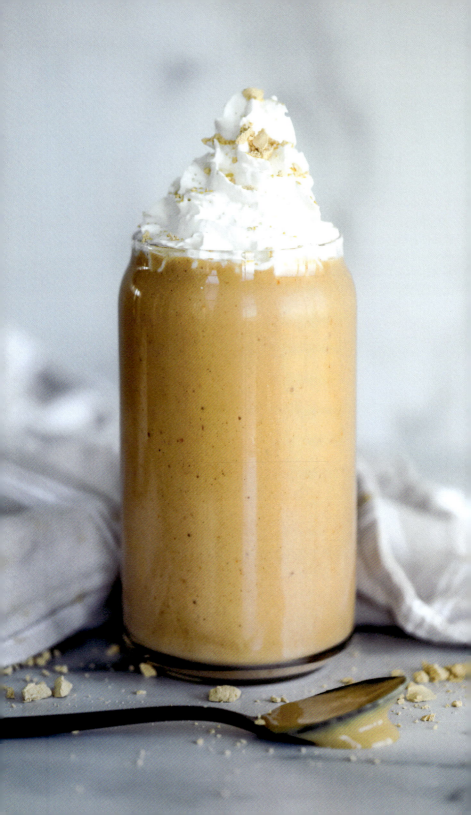

PB PUMPKIN CREAM SHAKE

Makes 1 serving
250 calories / 9F / 26C / 17P

1 cup unsweetened almond milk
½ serving (16g) CSE Simply Vanilla or Pumpkin Pie Protein Powder
50g frozen banana slices
¼ cup canned pumpkin
1 Tbs. powdered peanut butter
½ Tbs. OffBeat Sweet Classic Peanut Butter
   or natural peanut butter
½ tsp. pumpkin pie spice
8-10 (130g) ice cubes
Topping:
2 Tbs. spray whipped cream

1. Add all of the ingredients to a high-powered blender. Blend on high until smooth.

2. Pour into a cup, top with whipped cream and enjoy!

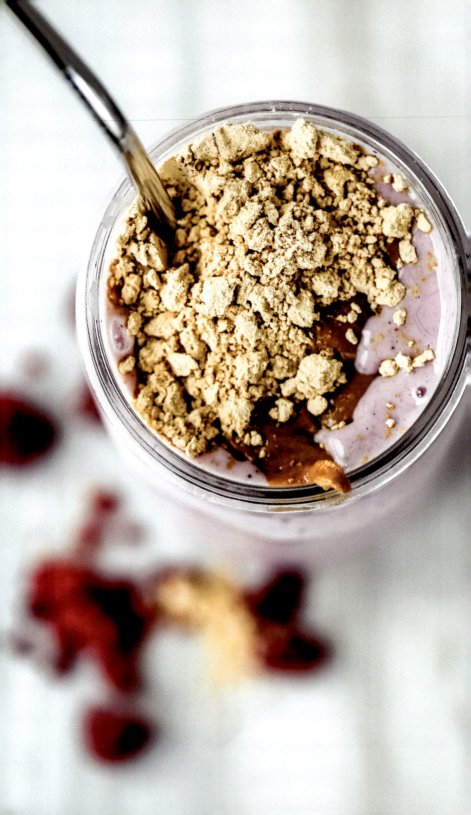

PB&J BREAKFAST SHAKE
Makes 1 serving
316 calories / 9.5F / 30C / 27.5P

1 cup unsweetened almond milk
1 serving CSE Simply Vanilla
   or Strawberry Cheesecake Protein Powder
5g CSE Super Berry Mix or 60g frozen berries
50g frozen banana slices
1 Tbs. OffBeat Sweet Classic Peanut Butter
   or natural peanut butter
¼ tsp. xanthan gum, to thicken
8-10 (130g) ice cubes
Topping:
1 Tbs. powdered peanut butter

1. Add all of the ingredients to a high-powered blender. Blend on high until smooth.

2. Pour into a cup. Top with powdered peanut butter and fold into the shake. Enjoy with a spoon or a thick straw.

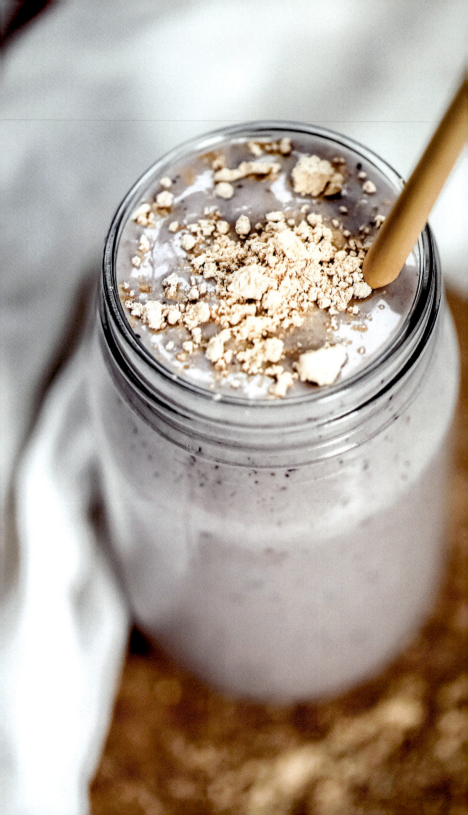

PB&J SNACK SHAKE

Makes 1 serving
240 calories / 8F / 23C / 19P

---

1 cup unsweetened almond milk
½ serving (16g) CSE Simply Vanilla
   or Strawberry Cheesecake Protein Powder
½ cup (70g) frozen berries of choice
30g frozen banana slices
1 Tbs. powdered peanut butter
½ Tbs. OffBeat Sweet Classic Peanut Butter
  or natural peanut butter
6-8 (120g) ice cubes

Topping:
1 Tbs. powdered peanut butter

1. Add all of the ingredients to a high-powered blender. Blend on high until smooth.

2. Pour into a cup, top with powdered peanut butter and enjoy!

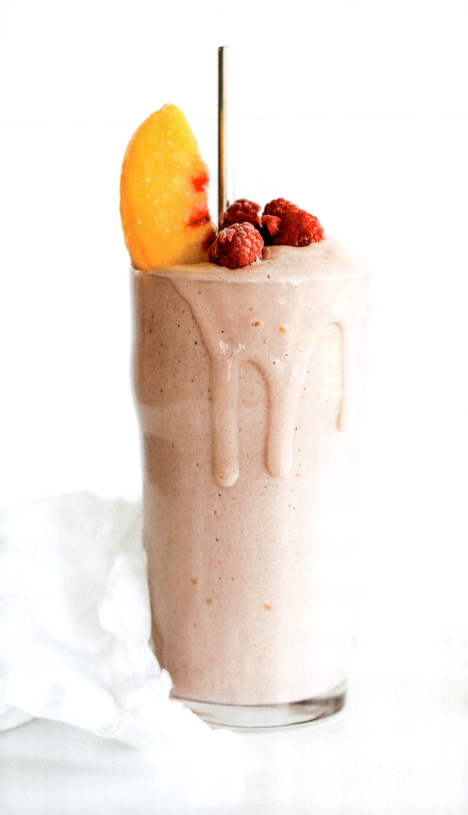

PEACH RASPBERRY COOLER (POST-WORKOUT)
Makes 1 serving
195 calories / 2F / 25C / 19P

---

1 cup unsweetened almond milk
¾ serving (24g) CSE Simply Vanilla
    or Strawberry Cheesecake Protein Powder
1 serving CSE Super Peach Mango Collagen Mix
1 serving CSE Super Berry Mix
20g frozen peaches
20g frozen raspberries
6-8 (120g) ice cubes

1. Add all of the ingredients to a high-powered blender. Blend on high until smooth.

2. Pour into a cup and enjoy after a workout!

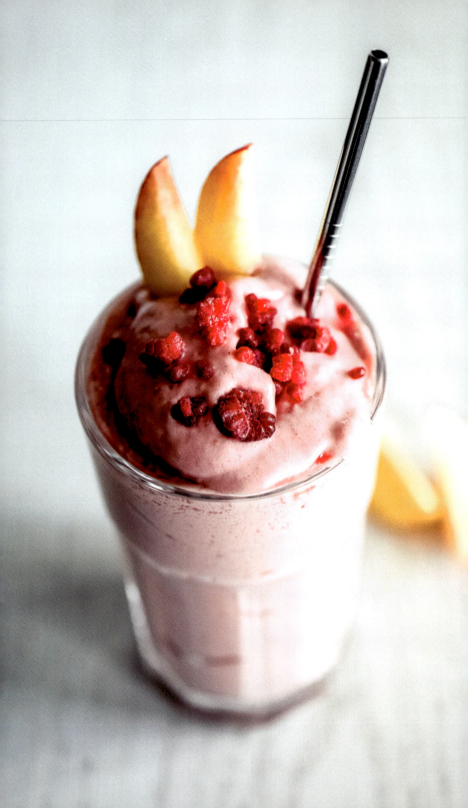

PEACH RASPBERRY SHAKE

Makes 1 serving
350 calories / 12F / 34.5C / 26.5P

1 cup unsweetened almond milk
½ cup low-fat cottage cheese
½ serving (16g) CSE Simply Vanilla Protein Powder
100g fresh, ripe peaches
100g frozen raspberries
30g avocado
Vanilla stevia drops
6-8 (100g) ice cubes

1. Add all of the ingredients to a high-powered blender. Blend on high until smooth.

2. Pour into a cup and enjoy after a workout!

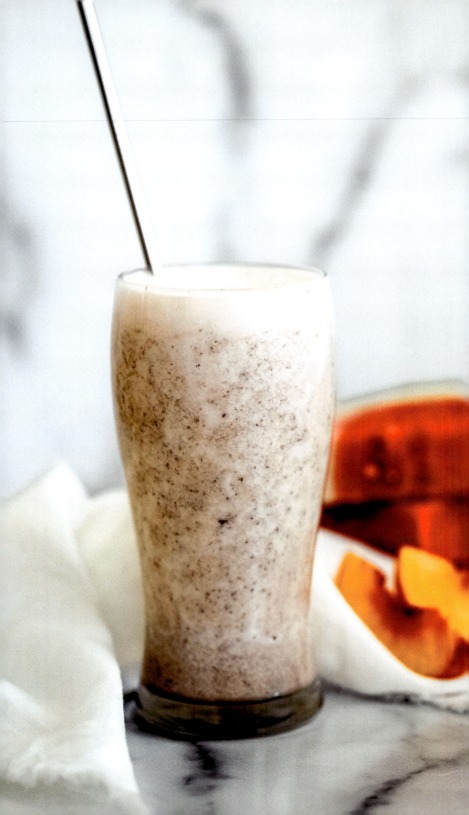

PEACH WATERMELON COOLER

Makes 1 serving
225 calories / 7F / 23C / 17P

½ cup lite canned coconut milk
50g fresh or frozen watermelon
50g fresh or frozen peaches
¾ serving (24g) CSE Simply Vanilla
    or Coconut Cream Protein Powder
1 tsp. chia seeds
6-8 (120g) ice cubes

1. Add all of the ingredients to a high-powered blender. Blend on high until smooth.

2. Pour into a cup and enjoy!

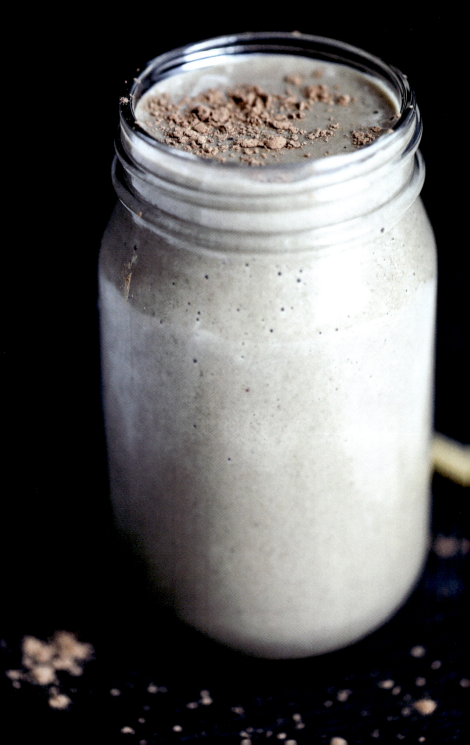

PEANUT BUTTER BROWNIE SHAKE

Makes 1 serving
240 calories / 7F / 25C / 21.5P

---

1 cup unsweetened almond milk
1 serving CSE Super Greens Mix
¾ serving (24g) CSE Brownie Batter
    or Chocolate Peanut Butter Protein Powder
1 Tbs. cocoa powder
45g frozen banana slices
½ Tbs. OffBeat Sweet Classic Peanut Butter,
    Buckeye Brownie Peanut Butter, or natural peanut butter
6-8 (120g) ice cubes

1. Add all of the ingredients to a high-powered blender. Blend on high until smooth.

2. Pour into a cup and enjoy!

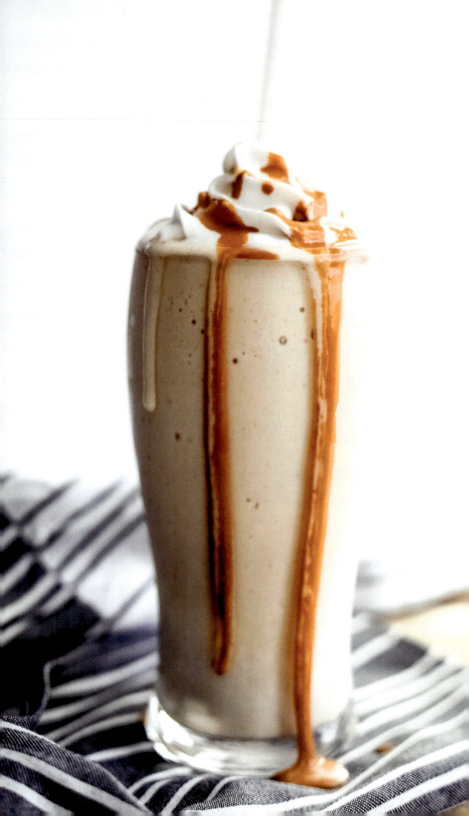

PEANUT BUTTER CARAMEL MILKSHAKE

Makes 1 serving
240 calories / 6.5F / 24C / 20.5P

½ cup fat-free milk
½ cup Vanilla Bean or Salted Caramel Halo Top Ice Cream
30g frozen banana slices
1 tsp. Walden Farms Caramel Syrup
2 Tbs. CSE Simply Vanilla Protein Powder
    or CSE Caramel Toffee Protein Powder
½ Tbs. OffBeat Sweet Classic Peanut Butter
    or natural peanut butter
6-8 (120g) ice cubes
Topping:
2 Tbs. spray whipped cream

1. Add all of the ingredients to a high-powered blender. Blend on high until smooth.

2. Pour into a cup, top with whipped cream and enjoy!

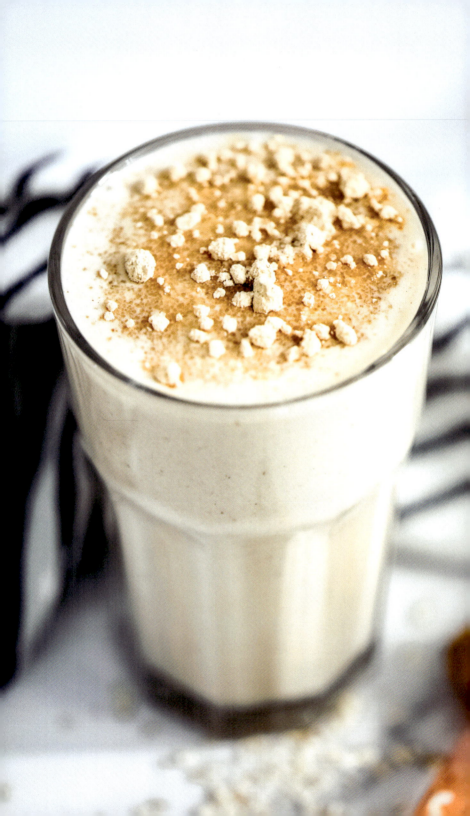

PEANUT BUTTER COOKIE BREAKFAST SHAKE

Makes 1 serving
335 calories / 9F / 33.5C / 30P

1 cup unsweetened almond milk
1 serving (32g) CSE Simply Vanilla Protein Powder
2 Tbs. old-fashioned rolled oats
40g frozen banana slices
2 Tbs. powdered peanut butter
1 Tbs. OffBeat Sweet Classic Peanut Butter
   or natural peanut butter
Dash sea salt
6-8 (120g) ice cubes
Topping:
1 tsp. sugar in the raw

1. Add all of the ingredients to a high-powered blender. Blend on high until smooth.

2. Sprinkle sugar in the raw on top. Enjoy!

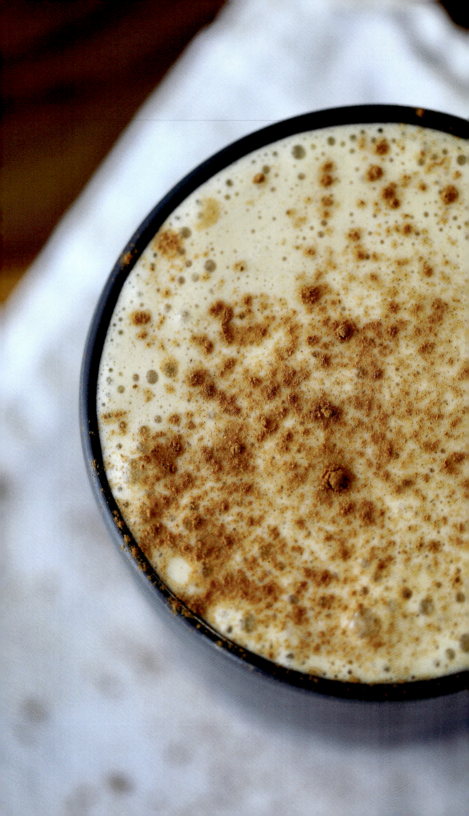

PEANUT BUTTER COOKIE SNACK SHAKE

Makes 1 serving
235 calories / 6.5F / 24.5C / 19P

1 cup unsweetened almond milk
½ serving (16g) CSE Simply Vanilla Protein Powder
2 Tbs. old-fashioned rolled oats
30g frozen banana slices
3 Tbs. powdered peanut butter
Dash cinnamon
6-8 (120g) ice cubes

1. Add all of the ingredients to a high-powered blender. Blend on high until smooth.

2. Pour into a cup and enjoy!

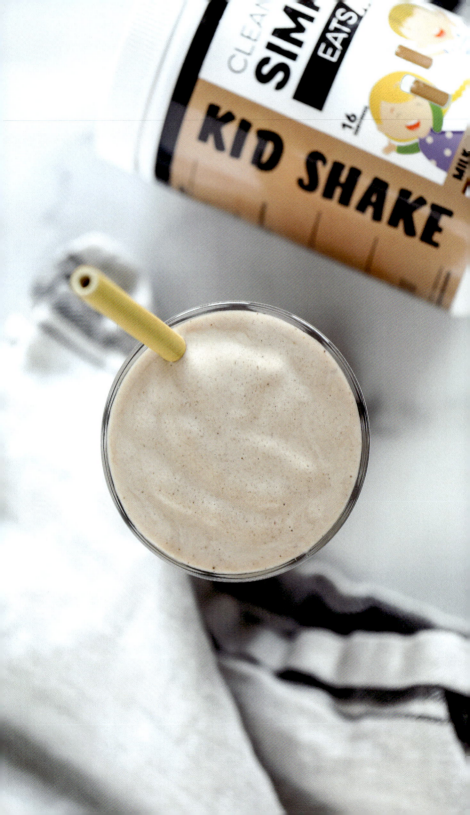

PEANUT BUTTER CUP SHAKE

Makes 1 serving
260 calories / 12F / 24C / 14P

---

1 cup unsweetened vanilla almond milk
1 serving CSE Milk Chocolate Kid Shake Protein Powder
40g frozen banana slices
1 Tbs. OffBeat Sweet Classic Peanut Butter
   or natural peanut butter
6-8 (120g) ice cubes

1. Add all of the ingredients to a high-powered blender. Blend on high until smooth.

2. Pour into a cup and enjoy!

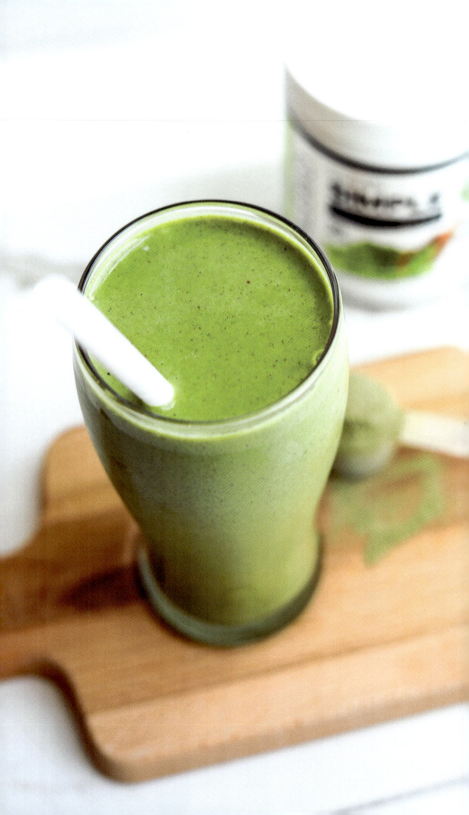

POWER GREENS SHAKE

Makes 1 serving
237 calories / 7F / 27C / 16P

---

1 cup unsweetened almond milk
¾ serving CSE Simply Vanilla Protein Powder
1 serving CSE Super Greens Mix
50g frozen banana slices
½ Tbs. OffBeat Aloha Butter, Almond Mocha Butter
   or natural almond butter
1 cup spinach
Dash of cinnamon
6-8 (120g) ice cubes

1. Add all of the ingredients to a high-powered blender. Blend on high until smooth.

2. Pour into a cup and enjoy!

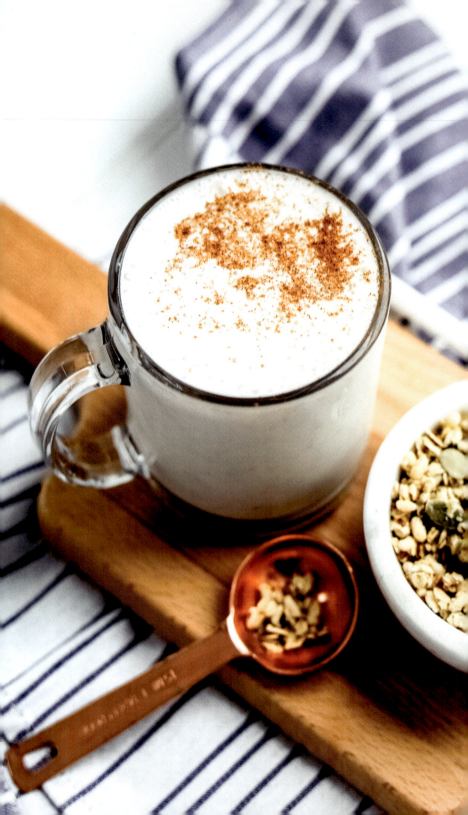

PROTEIN POWER CRUNCH SHAKE

Makes 1 serving
240 calories / 8F / 25C / 17P

---

1 cup unsweetened almond milk
½ cup low-fat cottage cheese
3 Tbs. Nature's Path Pumpkin Seed & Flax Granola
50g frozen banana slices
Dash cinnamon
Vanilla stevia drops, to taste
6-8 (120g) ice cubes

1. Add all of the ingredients to a high-powered blender. Blend on high until smooth.

2. Pour into a cup and enjoy!

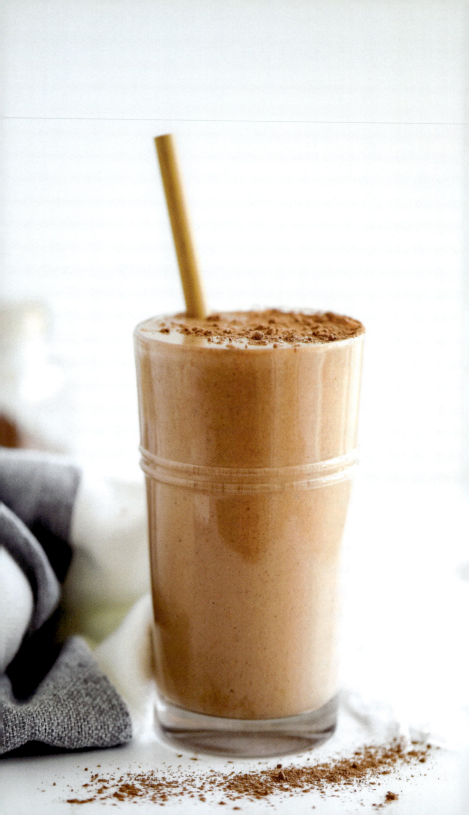

PUMPKIN COCOA SHAKE

Makes 1 serving
350 calories / 11.5F / 34C / 26.5P

1 cup unsweetened almond milk
1 serving CSE Brownie Batter Protein Powder
1 Tbs. cocoa powder
70g frozen banana slices
2 Tbs. canned pumpkin
1 Tbs. OffBeat Midnight Almond Coconut Butter
   or natural almond butter
Dash cinnamon
Dash pumpkin pie spice
6-8 (120g) ice cubes

1. Add all of the ingredients to a high-powered blender. Blend on high until smooth.

2. Pour into a cup and enjoy!

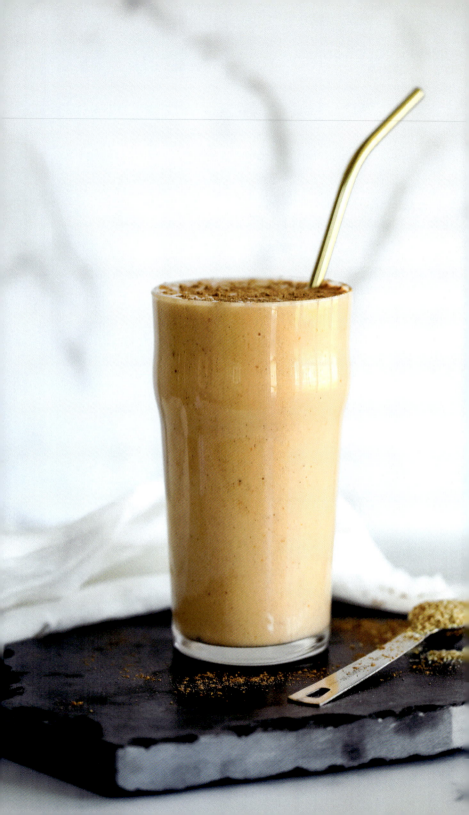

PUMPKIN SPICE SHAKE

Makes 1 serving
240 calories / 7.5F / 24C / 19P

1 cup unsweetened almond milk
¾ serving (24g) CSE Simply Vanilla
   or Pumpkin Pie Protein Powder
¼ cup canned pumpkin
40g frozen banana slices
½ Tbs. OffBeat Cinnamon Bun Butter, Pumpkin Spice Butter,
   or natural almond butter
1 tsp. flaxseed meal
Dash pumpkin pie spice
8-10 (130g) ice cubes

1. Add all of the ingredients to a high-powered blender. Blend on high until smooth.

2. Pour into a cup and enjoy!

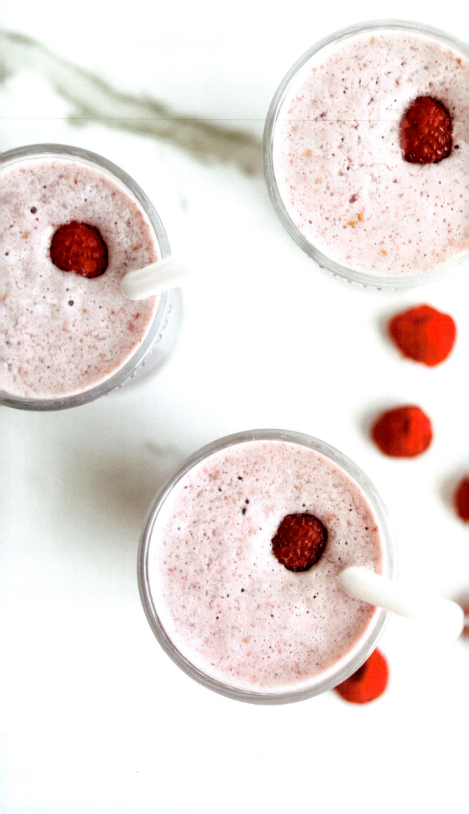

RADIANT RASPBERRY SHAKE

Makes 1 serving
210 calories / 7F / 23C / 16P

___

1 cup unsweetened almond milk
½ cup fresh or frozen raspberries
½ serving CSE Strawberry Cheesecake or Simply Vanilla
Protein Powder
1 serving CSE Super Berry Mix
2 Tbs. low-fat cottage cheese
½ Tbs. OffBeat Aloha Butter, Lemon Coconut Bliss Butter
   or natural almond butter
¼ tsp. almond extract
6-8 (120g) ice cubes

1. Add all of the ingredients to a high-powered blender. Blend on
high until smooth.

2. Pour into a cup and enjoy!

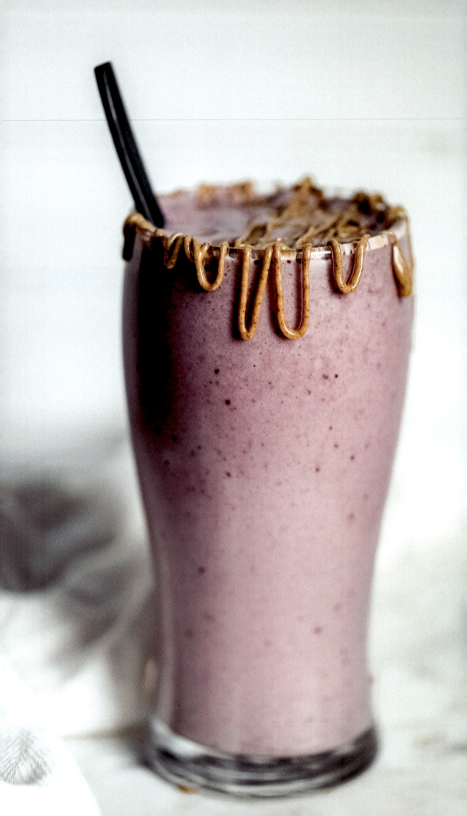

RASPBERRY MAPLE ALMOND SHAKE
Makes 1 serving
240 calories / 8.5F / 23.5C / 17P

---

1 cup unsweetened almond milk
75g frozen raspberries
40g frozen banana slices
½ serving (16g) CSE Simply Vanilla Protein Powder
2 Tbs. nonfat, plain Greek yogurt
¼-½ tsp. maple extract
8-10 (130g) ice cubes

Topping:
2 tsp. OffBeat Cinnamon Bun Butter, Salted Caramel Butter,
   or natural almond butter

1. Add all of the ingredients to a high-powered blender. Blend on high until smooth.

2. Pour into a cup, then drizzle the nut butter over the top. Enjoy!

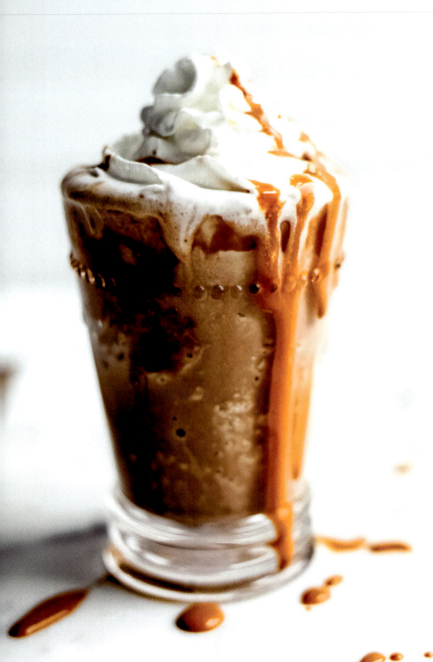

SNICKERS SHAKE

Makes 1 serving
220 calories / 7.5F / 22.5C / 16P

½ cup fat-free milk
2 Tbs. CSE Brownie Batter, Chocolate Peanut Butter,
   or Caramel Toffee Protein Powder
30g frozen banana slices
1 Tbs. old-fashioned rolled oats
2 tsp. OffBeat Sweet Classic Peanut Butter, Salted Caramel Butter,
   or natural peanut butter
1 tsp. cocoa powder
6-8 (120g) ice cubes
Topping:
2 Tbs. spray whipped cream
Walden Farms Caramel Syrup

1. Add all of the ingredients to a high-powered blender. Blend on high until smooth.

2. Pour into a cup. Top with whipped cream and caramel syrup. Enjoy!

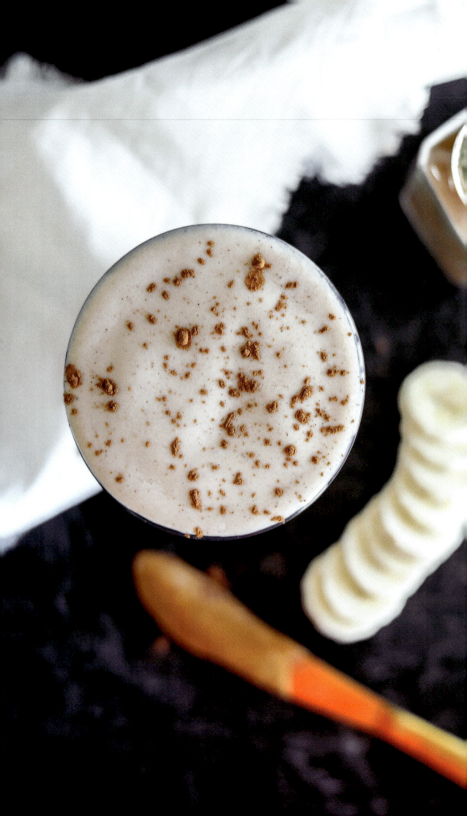

SPICED BANANA ALMOND SHAKE

Makes 1 serving
245 calories / 7F / 27.5C / 18.5P

---

1 cup unsweetened almond milk
¾ serving (24g) CSE Simply Vanilla, Bananas Foster,
    or Cinnamon Roll Protein Powder
½ Tbs. OffBeat Cinnamon Bun Butter
    or natural almond butter
80g frozen banana slices
¼ tsp. almond extract
Dash cinnamon
Dash nutmeg
8-10 (130g) ice cubes

1. Add all of the ingredients to a high-powered blender. Blend on
high until smooth.

2. Pour into a cup and enjoy!

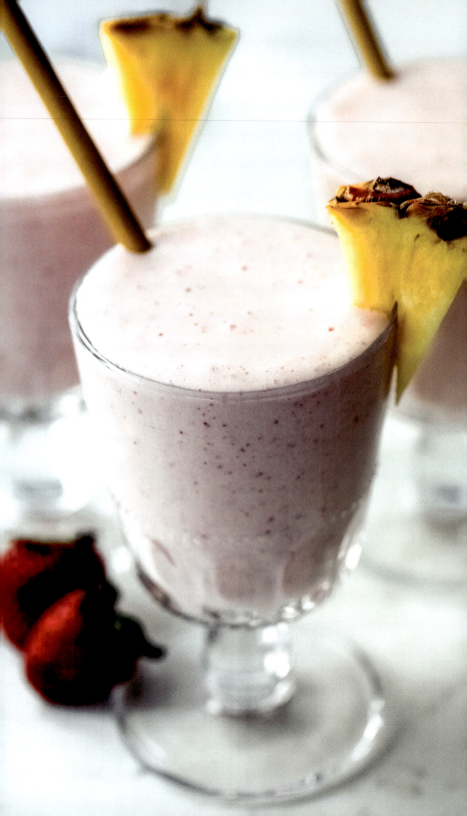

STRAWBERRY COLADA

Makes 1 serving
235 calories / 6F / 28C / 17P

½ cup lite canned coconut milk
½ serving (16g) CSE Simply Vanilla, Strawberry Cheesecake,
    or Coconut Cream Protein Powder
¼ cup nonfat, plain Greek yogurt
½ tsp. coconut extract
75g fresh or frozen strawberries
75g frozen pineapple
6-8 (120g) ice cubes

1. Add all of the ingredients to a high-powered blender. Blend on high until smooth.

2. Pour into a cup and enjoy!

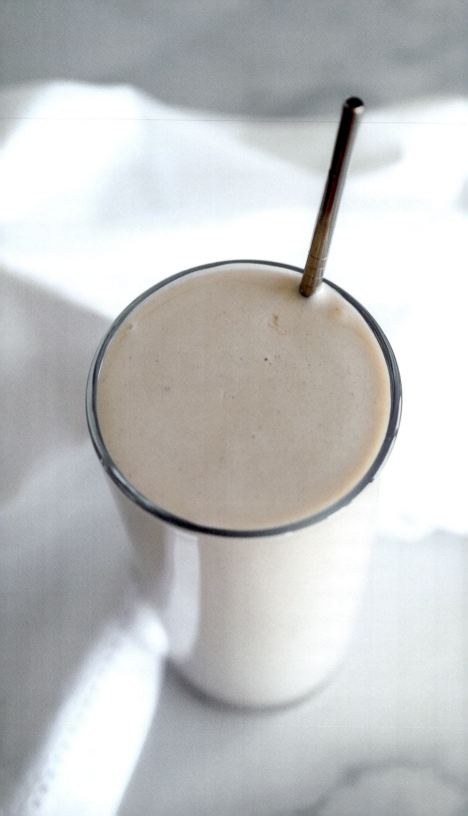

STRAWBERRY MILKSHAKE
(POST-WORKOUT)
Makes 1 serving
225 calories / 0F / 28C / 28P

---

1 cup fat-free milk
1 serving CSE Simply Vanilla
   or Strawberry Cheesecake Protein Powder
1 serving CSE Super Berry Mix
¼ tsp. xanthan gum, to thicken
8-10 (130g) ice cubes

1. Add all of the ingredients to a high-powered blender. Blend on high until smooth.

2. Pour into a cup and enjoy right after a workout.

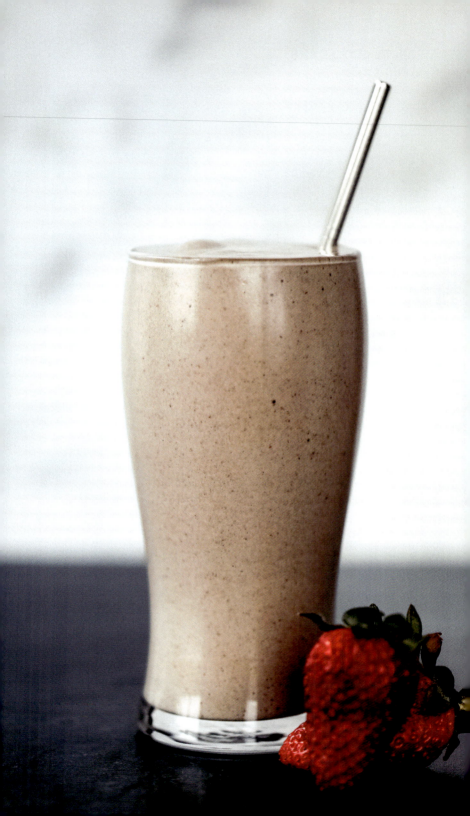

STRAWBERRY SUPER GREENS SMOOTHIE

Makes 1 serving
222 calories / 7F / 22.5C / 17.5P

---

1 cup unsweetened almond milk
¾ serving (24g) CSE Simply Vanilla
   or Strawberry Cheesecake Protein Powder
1 serving CSE Super Greens Mix
1 cup fresh or frozen strawberries
½ Tbs. OffBeat Butter of choice
   or natural almond butter
8-10 (130g) ice cubes

1. Add all of the ingredients to a high-powered blender and blend until smooth.

2. Pour into a cup and enjoy!

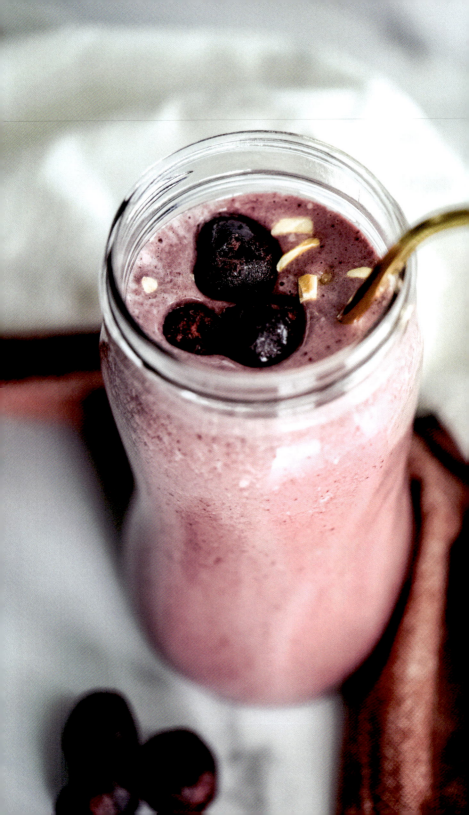

SWEET CHERRY ALMOND FREEZE
Makes 1 serving
350 calories / 13F / 32C / 26P

---

1 cup unsweetened almond milk
¼ cup nonfat, plain Greek yogurt
130g frozen, pitted, dark sweet cherries
¾ serving (24g) CSE Simply Vanilla
    or Brownie Batter Protein Powder
1 Tbs. OffBeat Almond Mocha Butter,
    Midnight Almond Coconut Butter or natural almond butter
½ tsp. almond extract
6-8 (120g) ice cubes

1. Add all of the ingredients to a high-powered blender. Blend on high until smooth.

2. Pour into a cup and enjoy!

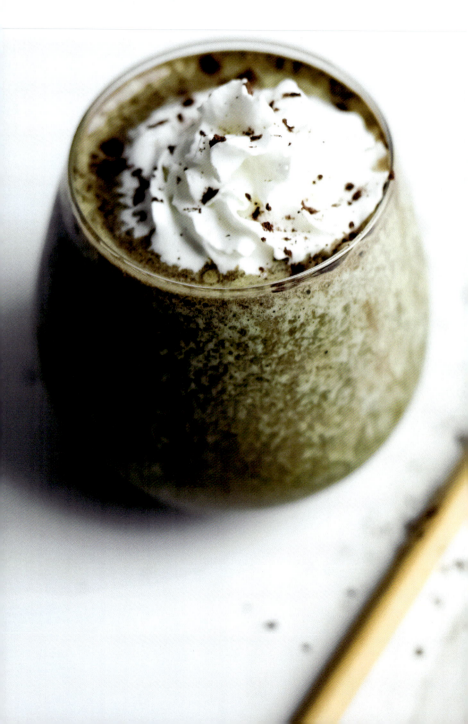

THIN MINT SHAKE
Makes 1 serving
240 calories / 9F / 24C / 15.5P

---

1 cup unsweetened almond milk
½ serving (17g) CSE Mint Chocolate Cookie
   or Brownie Batter Protein Powder
30g frozen banana slices
1 Tbs. OffBeat Mint Chocolate Chip Cookie Butter
1 Tbs. cocoa powder
1 cup spinach
6-8 (120g) ice cubes
Topping:
2 Tbs. spray whipped cream

1. Add all of the ingredients to a high-powered blender. Blend on high until smooth.

2. Top with whipped cream and enjoy!

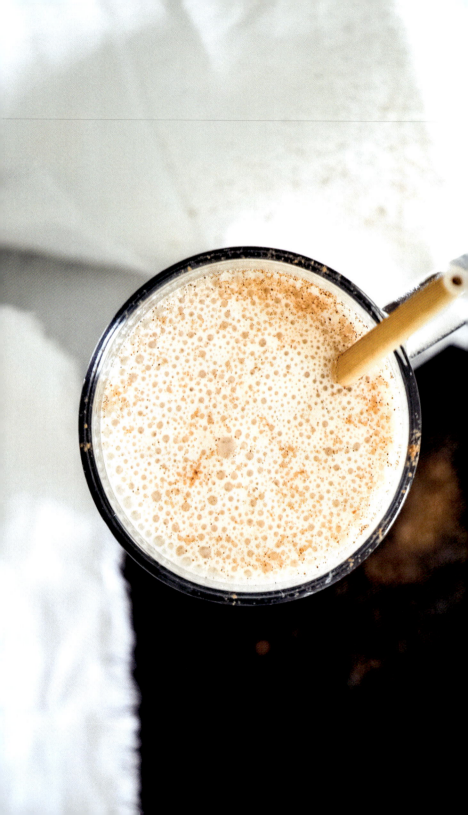

THOR-CHATA BREAKFAST SHAKE

Makes 1 serving
350 calories / 12.5F / 33C / 26P

---

1 cup unsweetened rice milk
1 serving CSE Simply Vanilla Protein Powder
2 Tbs. old-fashioned rolled oats
1 ½ Tbs. (21g) OffBeat Cinnamon Bun Butter
   or natural almond butter
½ tsp. vanilla paste or vanilla extract
½ tsp. ground cinnamon
6-8 (120g) ice cubes

1. Add all of the ingredients to a high-powered blender. Blend on high until smooth.

2. Pour into a cup and enjoy!

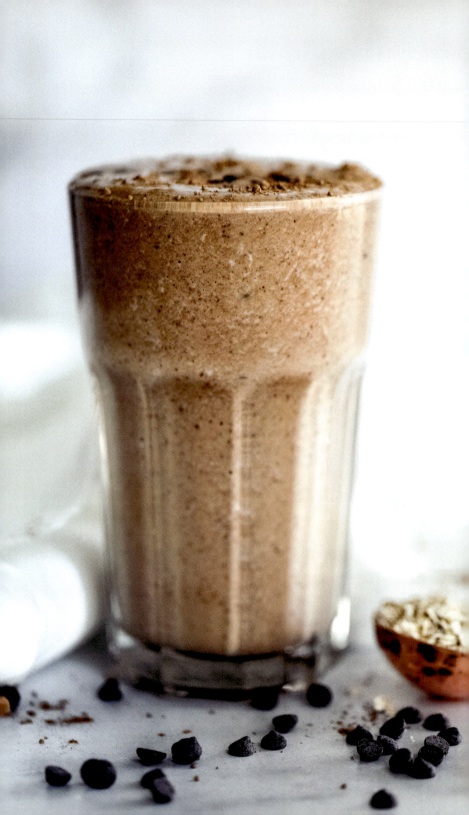

TRIPLE CHOCOLATE BROWNIE SHAKE

Makes 1 serving
330 calories / 10F / 35C / 24.5P

1 cup unsweetened vanilla almond milk
1 serving CSE Brownie Batter Protein Powder
30g frozen banana slices
2 Tbs. old-fashioned rolled oats
1 Tbs. cocoa powder
¼ tsp. vanilla extract
Dash sea salt
30 (15g) extra dark chocolate chips
6-8 (120g) ice cubes

1. Add all of the ingredients to a high-powered blender. Blend on high until smooth.

2. Pour into a cup and enjoy!

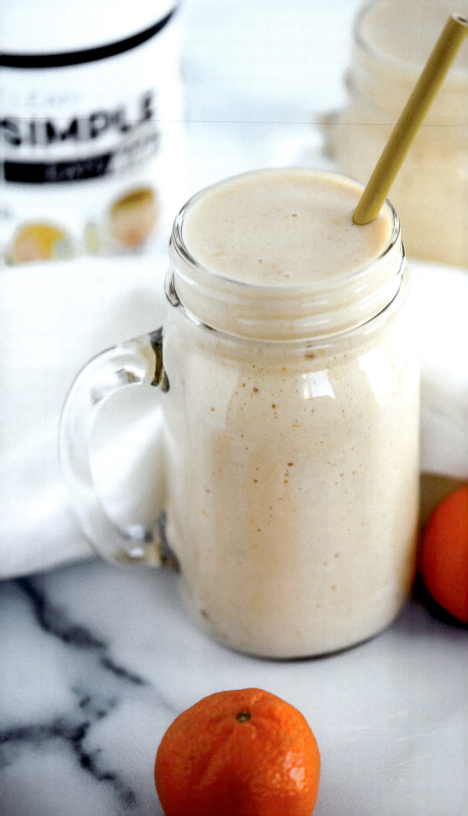

TROPICAL ORANGE SUNRISE SMOOTHIE

Makes 2 smoothies
195 calories / 2F / 29C / 15P / per smoothie

1 cup unsweetened vanilla almond milk
50g frozen bananas
120g frozen pineapple
120g clementine oranges
¼ cup low-fat cottage cheese
2 servings CSE Creamy Vanilla Kid Shake Protein Powder
6-8 (120g) ice cubes

1. Add all of the ingredients to a high-powered blender. Blend on high until smooth.

2. Pour into a cup and enjoy!

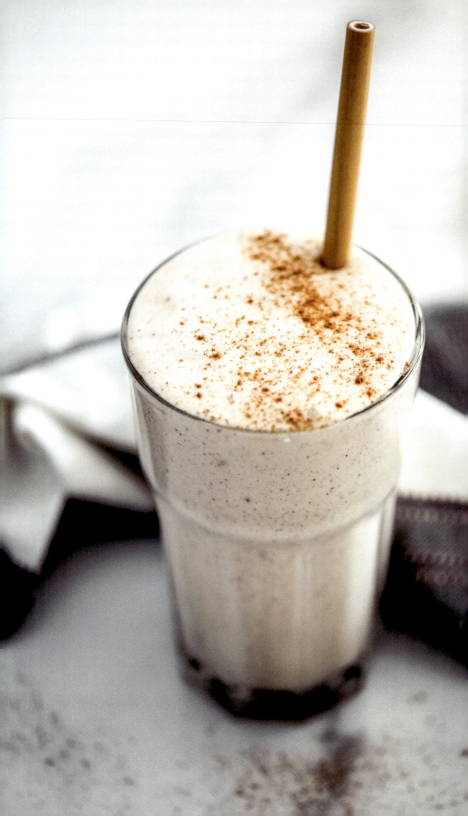

VANILLA CHAI SHAKE

Makes 1 serving
235 calories / 8.5F / 25C / 15P

---

1 cup unsweetened almond milk
½ serving (16g) CSE Simply Vanilla, Snickerdoodle,
   or Caramel Toffee Protein Powder
50g frozen banana slices
½ Tbs. OffBeat Cinnamon Bun Butter
   or natural almond butter
2 Tbs. old-fashioned rolled oats
1 tsp. chia seeds
1 tsp. ground cinnamon
¼ tsp. ground ginger
¼ tsp. cardamom
Dash cloves
6-8 (120g) ice cubes

1. Add all of the ingredients to a high-powered blender. Blend on high until smooth.

2. Pour into a cup and enjoy!

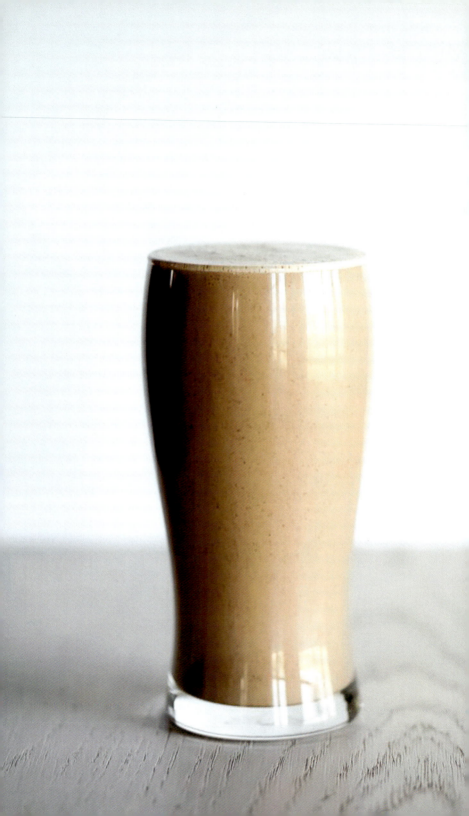

VEGAN DARK CHOCOLATE PEANUT BUTTER SHAKE

Makes 1 serving
345 calories / 12F / 34.5C / 25P

1 cup unsweetened almond milk
1 serving CSE Chocolate Vegan Protein Powder
100g frozen banana slices
1 Tbs. cocoa powder
1 Tbs. OffBeat Sweet Classic Peanut Butter
   or natural peanut butter
6-8 (120g) ice cubes

1. Add all of the ingredients to a high-powered blender. Blend on high until smooth.

2. Pour into a cup and enjoy!

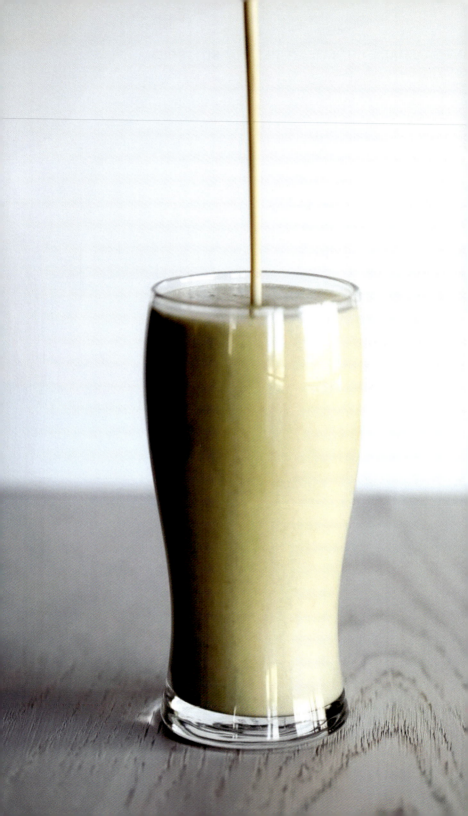

VEGAN VANILLA POWER SHAKE

Makes 1 serving
335 calories / 11.5F / 34C / 23.5P

---

1 cup unsweetened almond milk
1 serving CSE Vanilla Vegan Protein Powder
100g frozen banana slices
1 Tbs. OffBeat Butter of choice
    or natural almond butter
6-8 (120g) ice cubes

1. Add all of the ingredients to a high-powered blender. Blend on high until smooth.

2. Pour into a cup and enjoy!

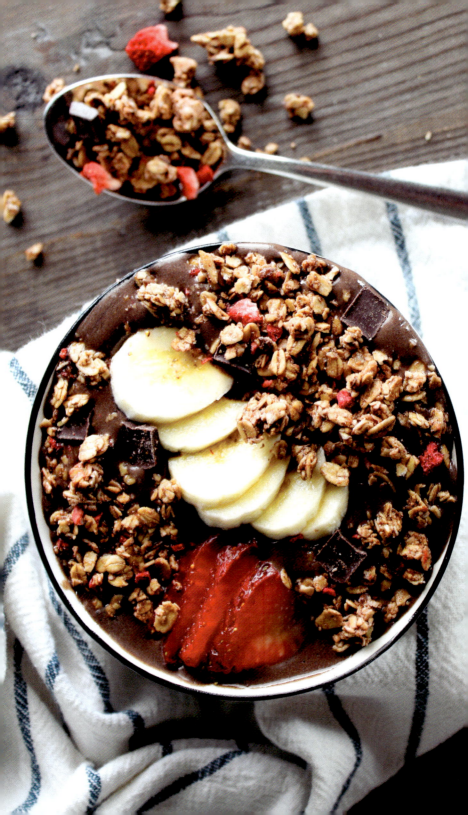

CHOCOLATE LOVER'S ACAI BOWL

Makes 1 serving
355 calories / 12F / 37C / 25P

1 frozen unsweetened Sambazon Açaí pack
¼ cup unsweetened almond coconut milk
40g frozen banana slices
1 serving CSE Brownie Batter Protein Powder
1 Tbs. special dark cocoa powder
4-6 (80g) ice cubes
Toppings:
20g banana slices
20g strawberry slices
1 Tbs. sliced almonds
1 Tbs. Dark Chocolate & Red Berries Love Crunch granola

1. Place frozen açaí in a blender and pulse until broken up. Scrape down the sides of the blender and add the almond coconut milk, frozen bananas, protein powder, cocoa powder and ice. Blend until smooth and thick.

2. Pour into a bowl and top with bananas, strawberries, almonds and granola.

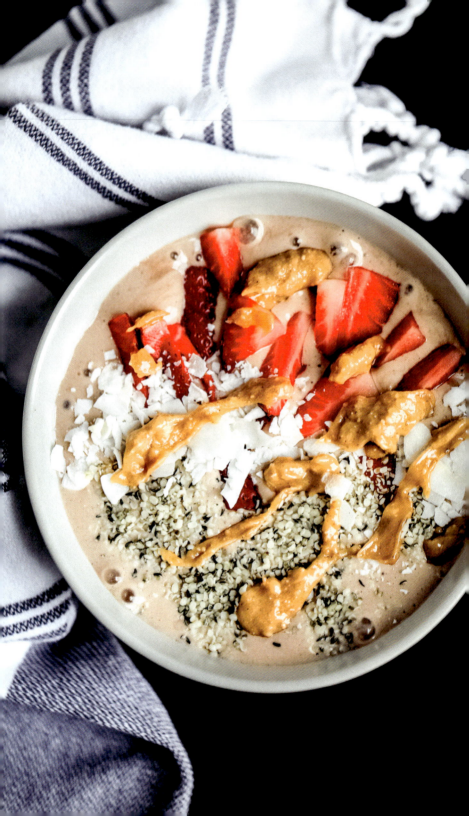

CHUNKY MONKEY SMOOTHIE BOWL

Makes 1 serving
250 calories / 9F / 25C / 19P

½ cup unsweetened almond milk
60g frozen banana slices
¾ serving (24g) CSE Brownie Batter
   or Chocolate Peanut Butter Protein Powder
¼ tsp. xanthan gum, optional to thicken
6-8 (120g) ice cubes

Toppings:
2 Tbs. berries of choice
½ Tbs. OffBeat Sweet Classic Peanut Butter,
   Monkey Business Butter, Candy Bar Butter,
   or natural peanut butter
½ Tbs. unsweetened shredded coconut
1 tsp. hemp seeds

1. Add all of the ingredients to a high-powered blender. Blend on high until smooth.

2. Pour into a bowl and top with with berries, coconut, hemp seeds and peanut butter. Enjoy with a spoon.

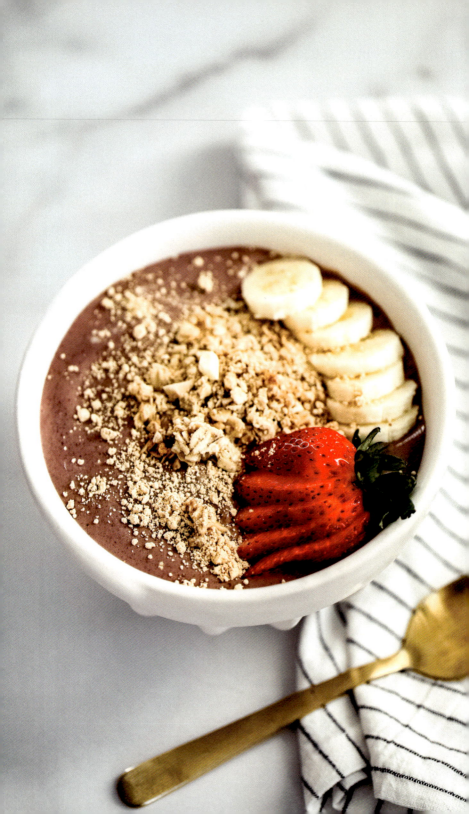

NUTTY BUTTER ACAI BOWL

Makes 1 serving
355 calories / 12F / 35C / 27P

---

1 frozen unsweetened Sambazon Açaí pack
40g frozen bananas
¼ cup unsweetened almond coconut milk
1 serving CSE Simply Vanilla Protein Powder
½ Tbs. OffBeat Sweet Classic Peanut Butter
   or natural peanut butter
4-6 (80g) ice cubes

Toppings:
20g banana, sliced
20g strawberries, sliced
1 Tbs. granola
1 tsp. powdered peanut butter

1. Place frozen açaí in a blender and pulse until broken up. Scrape down the sides of the blender and add the almond coconut milk, frozen bananas, protein powder, peanut butter and ice. Blend until smooth and thick.

2. Pour into a bowl and top with bananas, strawberries, granola and powdered peanut butter.

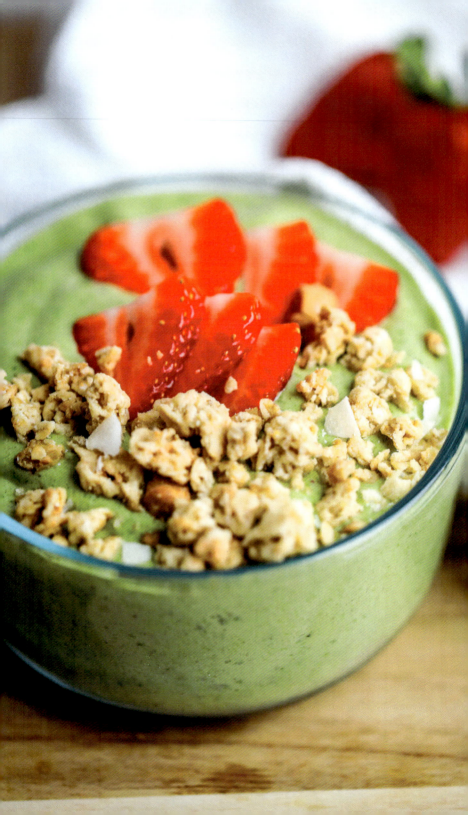

SUPER GREENS SMOOTHIE BOWL

Makes 1 serving
342 calories / 12.5F / 36C / 20P

½ cup unsweetened almond coconut milk
1 cup chopped spinach
60g frozen banana slices
1 Tbs. OffBeat Aloha Butter
   or natural almond butter
½ serving (5g) CSE Super Greens Mix
1 serving CSE Simply Vanilla or Coconut Cream Protein Powder
¼ tsp. xanthan gum, to thicken
6-8 (120g) ice cubes

Toppings:
30g sliced strawberries
10g Nature's Path Coconut & Cashew Butter granola

1. Add the almond coconut milk, spinach, banana slices, nut butter, Super Greens Mix, protein powder, xanthan gum, and ice to a high-powered blender. Blend until thick and smooth.

2. Pour into a bowl. Top with sliced strawberries and granola. Enjoy with a spoon.

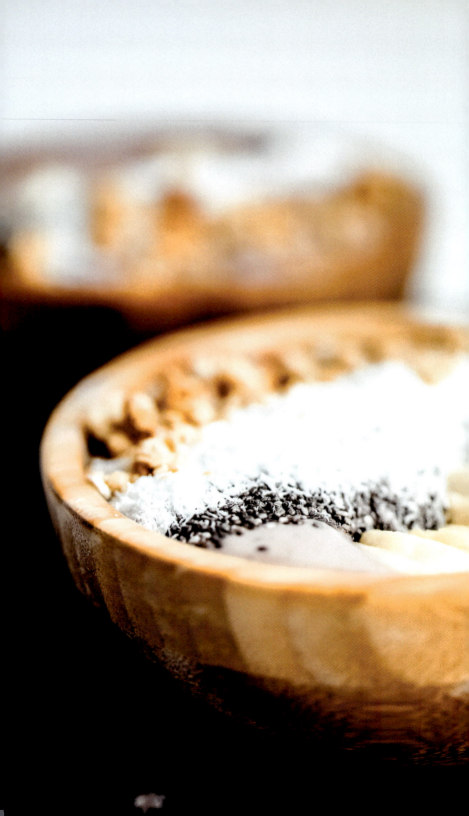

THE ORIGINAL ACAI BOWL
Makes 2 servings
240 calories / 8F / 25.5C / 16P / per serving

1 frozen unsweetened Sambazon Açaí pack
¼ cup unsweetened almond coconut milk
50g frozen strawberries
40g frozen banana slices
1 ¼ servings (40g) CSE Simply Vanilla Protein Powder
¼ tsp. xanthan gum, to thicken
4-6 (80g) ice cubes
Toppings per serving:
20g banana slices
1 Tbs. Nature's Path Coconut & Cashew Butter granola
½ tsp. unsweetened shredded coconut
½ tsp. chia seeds

1. Place frozen açaí in a blender and pulse until broken up. Scrape down the sides of the blender and add the almond milk, frozen strawberries, frozen banana slices, protein powder and ice cubes. Blend until smooth and thick.

2. Pour evenly into two bowls and top with banana slices, granola, coconut and chia seeds. Enjoy!

BROWNIES, COOKIES & BARS

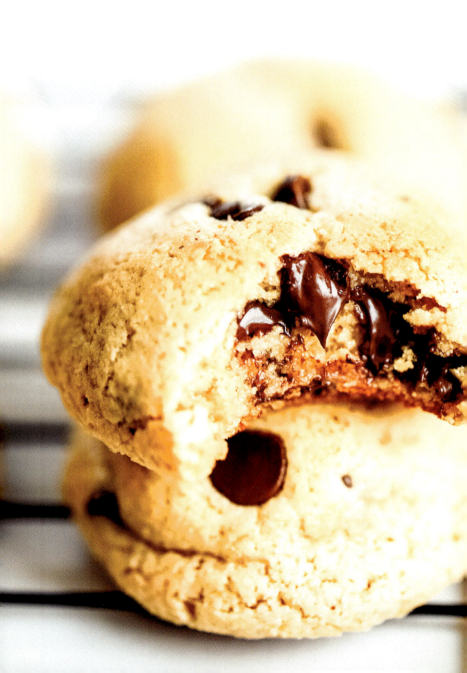

COOKIES MAKE EVERYTHING BETTER

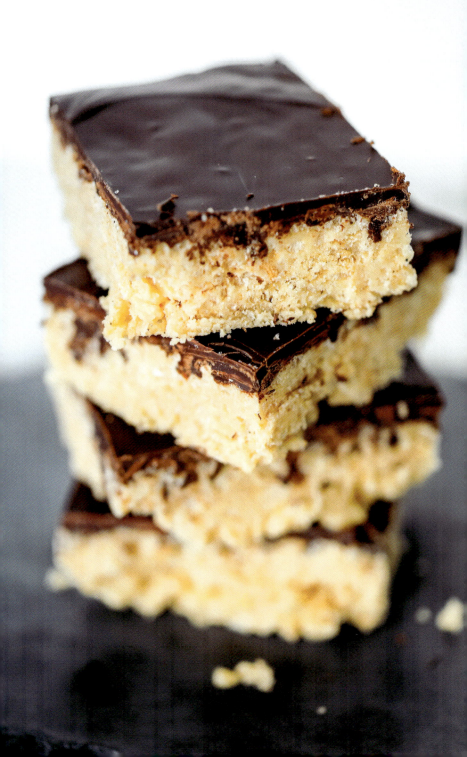

CHOCOLATE COVERED ALOHA BARS
Makes 20 bars
255 calories / 15F / 26C / 4P / per bar

Bars:
12 oz. OffBeat Aloha Butter
   or coconut butter
1 Tbs. coconut oil or grass-fed butter
½ cup raw honey
1 serving CSE Simply Vanilla or Coconut Cream Protein Powder
4 cups crispy rice cereal
Topping:
12 oz. dark chocolate chips
1 tsp. coconut oil

1. Add the Aloha Butter, coconut oil or butter and honey to a small saucepan. Heat over low/medium heat and stir constantly until melted down and pourable. Remove from heat and whisk in the protein powder.

2. Pour the crispy rice cereal into a large bowl. Pour the hot mixture over the top of the cereal and beat together until well combined. Press the mixture into a greased 9x13 pan.

3. Add the dark chocolate chips and coconut oil to a small saucepan over low/medium heat. Stir constantly until melted and smooth.

4. Pour the melted chocolate over the bars in the pan and spread out until smooth. Place in the fridge for about 2 hours or until the chocolate has hardened. Remove from the fridge and let soften about 10 minutes before cutting. Cut into 20 squares and serve. Store leftovers in the fridge.

*Swap in any flavor of OffBeat Butter for a different variety of bar.

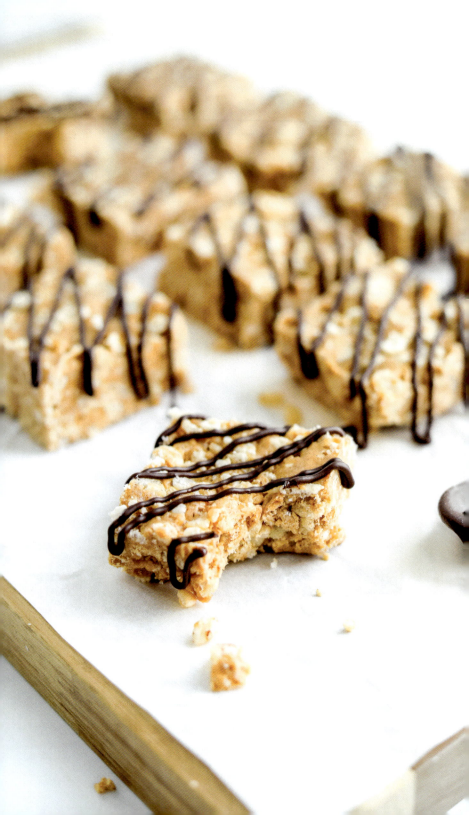

CRISPY CARAMEL BUTTERSCOTCH BARS

Makes 18 bars
225 calories / 12.5F / 23C / 5P / per bar

Bars:
12 oz. OffBeat Salted Caramel Butter
  or natural almond butter
½ cup raw honey
2 Tbs. unsweetened almond milk
½ cup butterscotch chips
1 serving CSE Caramel Toffee Protein Powder
3 ¾ cups crispy rice cereal
Topping:
¼ cup dark chocolate chips

1. Add the nut butter, honey, almond milk and butterscotch chips to a saucepan over low/medium heat. Stir until the butterscotch chips are melted and the mixture is smooth. Remove from heat and stir in the protein powder. Mix until well combined.

2. Pour the cereal into a large bowl and top with the caramel butterscotch mixture. Beat together until the ingredients are well combined. Press into a greased 9x13 pan. Store in the fridge until hardened and cool.

3. Place the chocolate chips in a small bowl. Microwave for 1-2 minutes or until melted and smooth, stirring every 30 seconds.

4. Remove the bars from the 9x13 pan onto a cutting board. Cut into 18 squares. Drizzle the chocolate over the top of the bars. Let the chocolate harden, then enjoy! Store leftovers in the fridge.

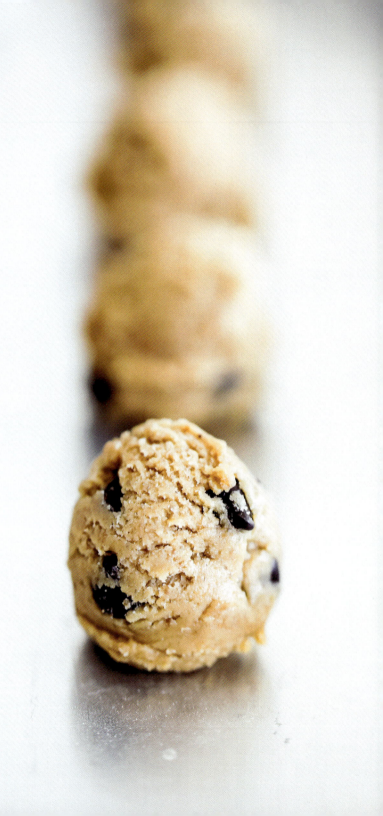

EDIBLE CHOCOLATE CHIP COOKIE DOUGH

Makes 16 cookies
155 calories / 9F / 18C / 2.5P / per cookie

½ cup softened grass-fed butter
½ cup coconut sugar
⅓ cup xylitol natural sweetener
¼ cup pasteurized liquid egg whites
1 tsp. vanilla extract
1 ½ cups old-fashioned rolled oats or oat flour
¼ tsp. sea salt
3 oz. dark chocolate chips

1. Add the butter, coconut sugar and xylitol to a bowl. Beat until smooth. Add in the egg whites and vanilla. Beat until combined.

2. Add in the oat flour, sea salt and chocolate chips. Mix on low until well combined.

3. Using a cookie scoop, scoop into cookie dough balls. Place in a container and store in the fridge or freezer. Stays fresh 2 weeks in the fridge and up to 3 months in the freezer.

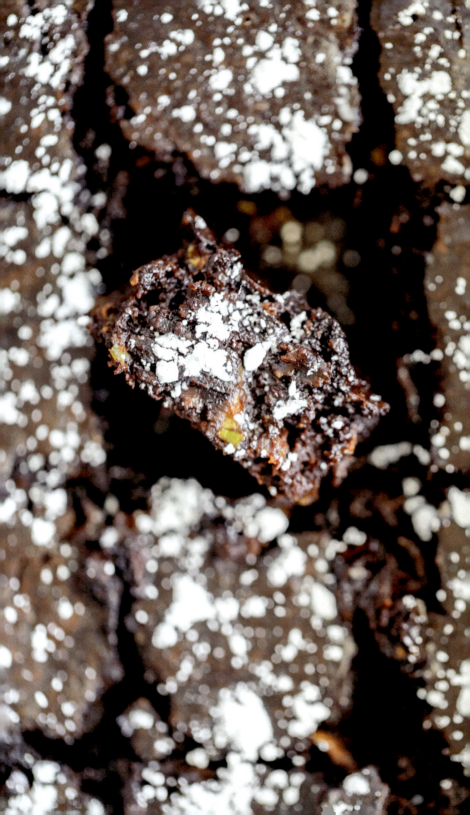

FLOURLESS ZUCCHINI BROWNIES

Makes 16 brownies
205 calories / 13F / 18C / 4P / per brownie

---

1 ½ cups peeled and grated zucchini
1 large egg
1 cup natural almond butter
⅓ cup raw honey
⅓ cup unsweetened applesauce
⅓ cup cocoa powder
2 Tbs. coconut sugar
1 tsp. vanilla extract
1 tsp. baking powder
Topping:
1 cup (180g) dark chocolate chips

1. Preheat the oven to 350 degrees.

2. Peel and grate the zucchini. Squeeze out most of the moisture; set aside.

3. Add all of the other ingredients to a large bowl and beat until well combined. Fold the zucchini into the batter.

4. Pour the batter into a greased 9x13 baking pan. Sprinkle the chocolate chips over the top and bake for 28-30 minutes. Let cool and cut into 16 squares. Enjoy!

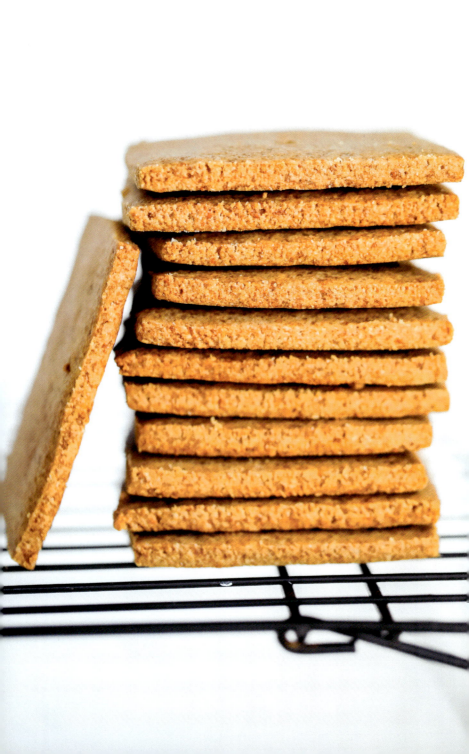

HOMEMADE GRAHAM COOKIES
Makes 12 cookies
100 calories / 5F / 14.5C / 1P / per cookie

¼ cup melted coconut oil
¼ cup coconut sugar
2 Tbs. raw honey
2 Tbs. water
½ tsp. vanilla extract
1 cup whole wheat pastry flour
½ tsp. cinnamon
½ tsp. baking soda

1. Preheat the oven to 350 degrees.

2. Add the melted coconut oil, coconut sugar and raw honey to a bowl. Beat until well combined. Add the water and vanilla, then beat until smooth.

3. Add the flour, cinnamon and baking soda to a separate bowl. Stir until combined. Add the dry ingredients to the wet ingredients and mix until well combined.

4. Place the dough on a large piece of parchment paper. Lightly flour a rolling pin with extra whole wheat pastry flour. Roll the dough out into a rectangular shape. Slice into 12 squares and place on a baking sheet. Bake for 10-15 minutes. Let cool on baking sheet for 2 minutes, then transfer to a cooling rack. Enjoy!

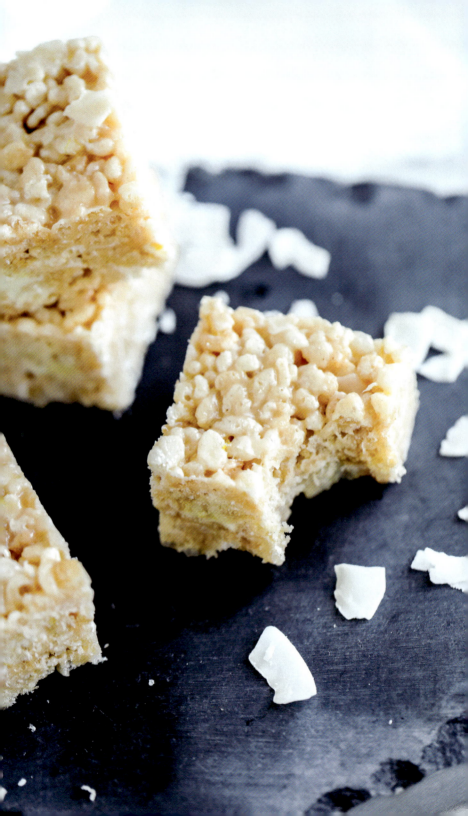

LEMON-BERRY COCONUT KRISPIES

Makes 16 servings
135 calories / 7.5F / 16C / 1.5P / per serving

4 Tbs. grass-fed butter
2 Tbs. raw honey
½ cup OffBeat Lemon Coconut Bliss Butter
   or coconut butter
16 Strawberries & Cream Smashmallows
4 cups crispy rice cereal
¼ cup unsweetened flaked coconut
2 Tbs. white chocolate chips
1 tsp. lemon zest

1. In a large saucepan melt the butter, honey and coconut butter over low heat. Add the marshmallows and stir until completely melted. Remove from heat.

2. Add the crispy rice cereal, flaked coconut, white chocolate chips and lemon zest to the saucepan. Stir until well coated.

3. Press the mixture into a greased 8x8 baking pan. Let cool, then cut into squares.

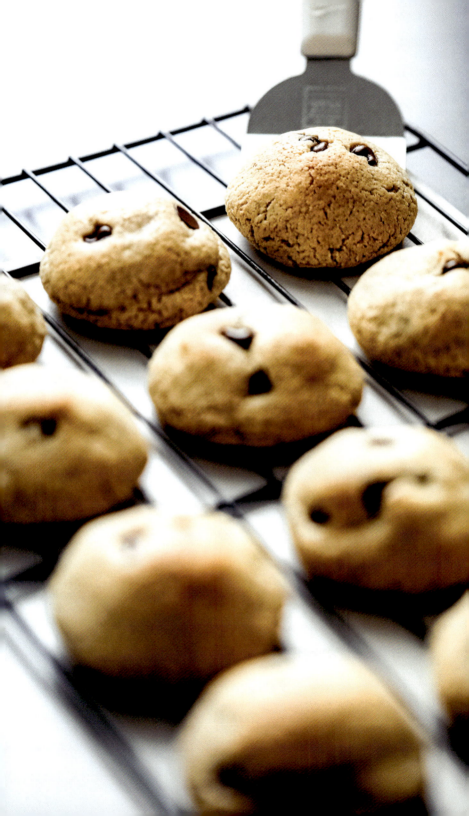

PROTEIN PEANUT BUTTER COOKIES

Makes 26 cookies
160 calories / 10F / 11.5C / 7.5P / per cookie

---

1 cup OffBeat Sweet Classic Peanut Butter
   or natural peanut butter
½ cup xylitol natural sweetener
½ cup raw honey
2 large eggs
1 Tbs. vanilla extract
2 servings CSE Simply Vanilla Protein Powder
2 cups almond flour
1 tsp. sea salt
1 tsp. baking soda
½ tsp. baking powder
½ cup dark chocolate chips

1. Heat oven to 350 degrees.

2. Add the peanut butter, xylitol and raw honey to a bowl. Beat together until creamy. Add in the eggs and vanilla. Beat until well combined.

3. In a separate bowl, add the protein powder, almond flour, sea salt, baking soda and baking powder. Stir until combined. Add the dry mixture to the wet mixture and mix until just combined. Fold in the chocolate chips.

4. Using a large cookie scoop, scoop the cookie dough onto a baking sheet lined with parchment paper. Cook time 7-9 minutes. Let cool on the pan for 2 minutes, then transfer to a cooling rack. Store leftovers in the fridge.

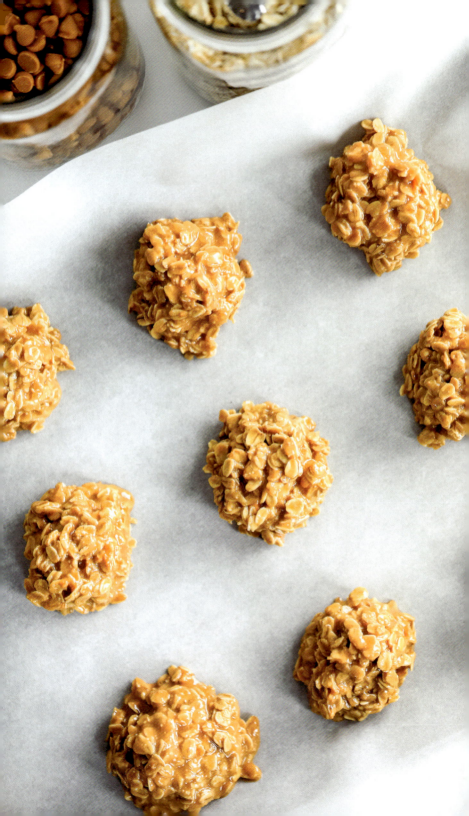

SALTED CARAMEL NO-BAKE COOKIES

Makes 12 cookies
350 calories / 21F / 33C / 6.5P / per cookie

¾ cup xylitol natural sweetener
¼ cup grass-fed butter
¼ cup unsweetened vanilla almond milk
¾ cup OffBeat Salted Caramel Butter
   or natural almond butter
½ cup butterscotch chips or dark chocolate chips
2 cups old-fashioned rolled oats

1. Line a baking sheet with wax or parchment paper.

2. Add the xylitol, butter and almond milk to a pot over medium heat, stirring constantly. Bring to a boil for 1 minute and remove from heat. Stir in the Salted Caramel Butter, butterscotch or dark chocolate chips and rolled oats.

3. Drop spoonfuls of the mixture onto the baking sheet and let sit about 30-60 minutes until hardened, or speed it up by cooling in the fridge. Enjoy!

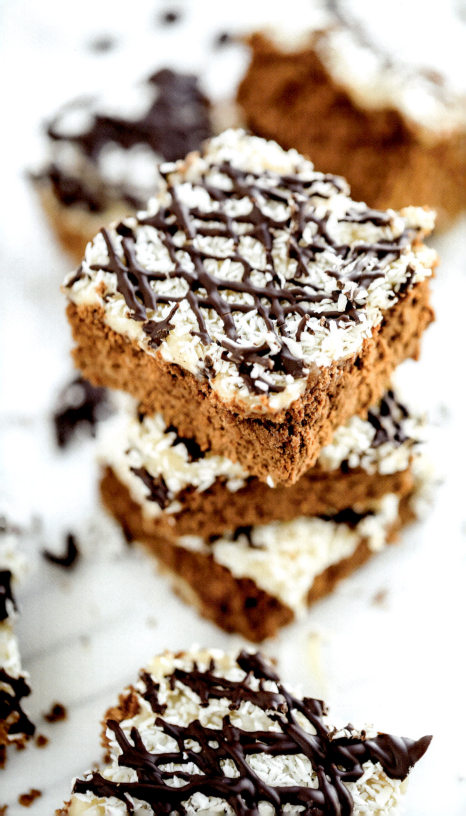

SAMOAS BROWNIES

Makes 16 brownies
300 calories / 15F / 40.5C / 4.5P / per brownie

Brownies:
¼ cup grass-fed butter
1 cup xylitol natural sweetener
¼ cup unsweetened applesauce
2 Tbs. pure maple syrup
6 Tbs. dutch-processed cocoa powder
½ serving (17g) CSE Brownie Batter Protein Powder
½ tsp. baking powder
¼ tsp. sea salt
¾ cup whole wheat pastry flour
2 large eggs
2 tsp. vanilla extract

Toppings:
1 recipe Cashew Coconut Caramel Sauce (recipe on page 147)
½ cup unsweetened shredded coconut
½ cup dark chocolate chips

1. Prepare the Cashew Coconut Caramel Sauce; set aside.

2. Add the butter to a medium-sized saucepan and melt down over low/medium heat. Once melted, whisk in the xylitol, applesauce and maple syrup until dissolved. Remove from the heat.

3.. Pour into a mixing bowl and add the cocoa powder, protein powder, baking powder, sea salt and flour. Mix until well combined. Beat in the eggs and vanilla last.

4. Pour batter into a greased 9x13 baking dish. Bake for 12-15 minutes. Should still be slightly gooey. Let cool completely before adding the toppings.

5. Pour the caramel sauce onto the cooled brownies and spread out evenly. Sprinkle the shredded coconut and chocolate chips over the top and press into the caramel sauce with the back of a spatula. Slice and enjoy!

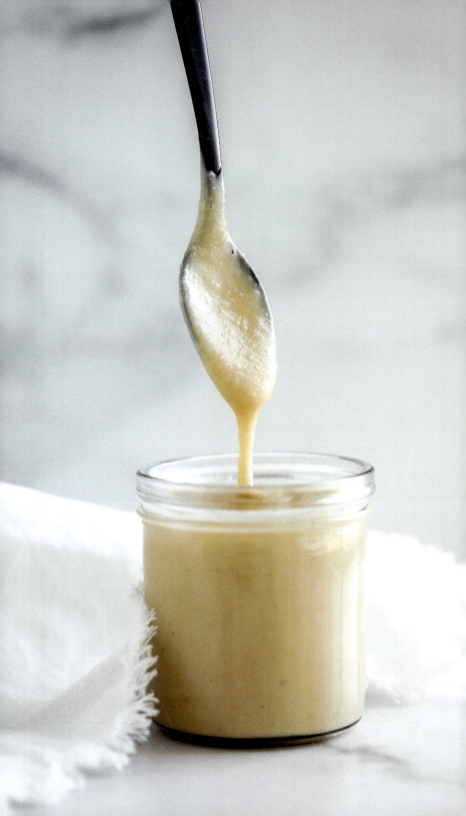

CASHEW COCONUT CARAMEL SAUCE

Makes 16 servings
130 calories / 7F / 16C / 1.5P / per serving

¾ cup salted cashews
¾ cup raw honey
½ cup unsweetened coconut flakes
2-3 Tbs. water
½ tsp. caramel or vanilla extract

1. Soak cashews in water for 1 hour.

2. Drain the cashews. Place in a high-powered blender with the rest of the ingredients and blend until smooth.

3. Weigh the sauce and divide the weight by 16 to get the amount needed to fill one serving. Store in the fridge until ready to use.

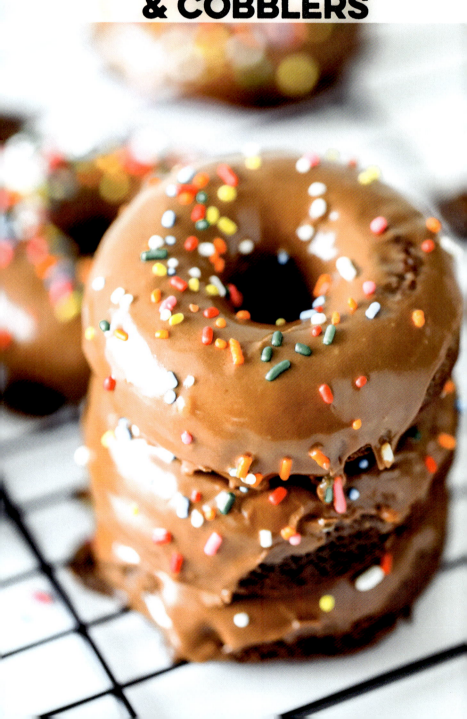

DONUT EVER GIVE UP.

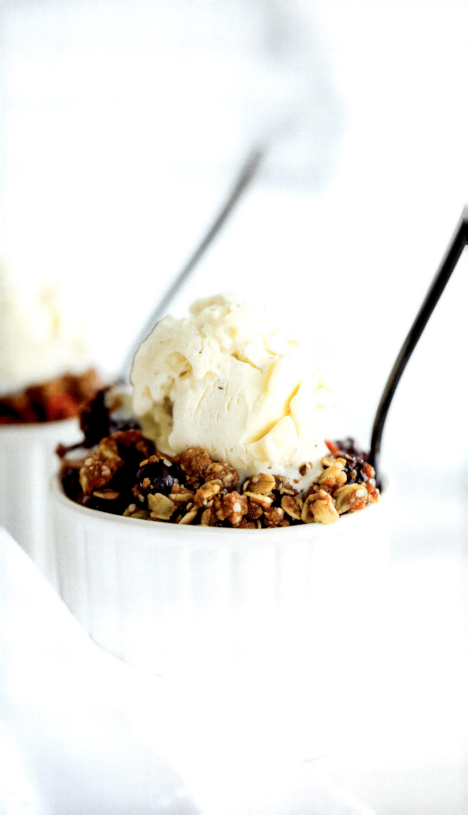

BERRY COBBLER CRUMBLE

Makes 15 servings
290 calories / 13.5F / 37.5C / 4.5P / per serving

---

2 cups blueberries
2 cups blackberries
2 cups raspberries
¼ cup raw honey
2 cups old-fashioned rolled oats
1 cup whole wheat pastry flour
½ cup hemp seed hearts
1 cup coconut sugar
2 tsp. cinnamon
½ tsp. nutmeg
1 cup melted grass-fed butter or coconut oil
Optional toppings:
Spray whipped cream
High protein ice cream

1. Preheat the oven to 350 degrees.

2. Add the berries and honey to a large bowl. Stir together until the berries are well coated in the honey. Set aside.

3. In a separate bowl add the oats, flour, hemp hearts, coconut sugar, cinnamon and nutmeg. Whisk together. Add the melted butter or coconut oil and stir until well combined and crumbly.

4. Press ⅔ of the crumble mixture into the bottom of a greased 9x13 baking dish. Pour the berry mixture and all the juices from the bowl over the crust. Top evenly with the remaining crumble mixture.

5. Bake for 30-35 minutes. Serve warm. Top each individual serving with vanilla high protein ice cream or spray whipped cream. Store leftovers in the fridge.

*Toppings not included in macros listed above.

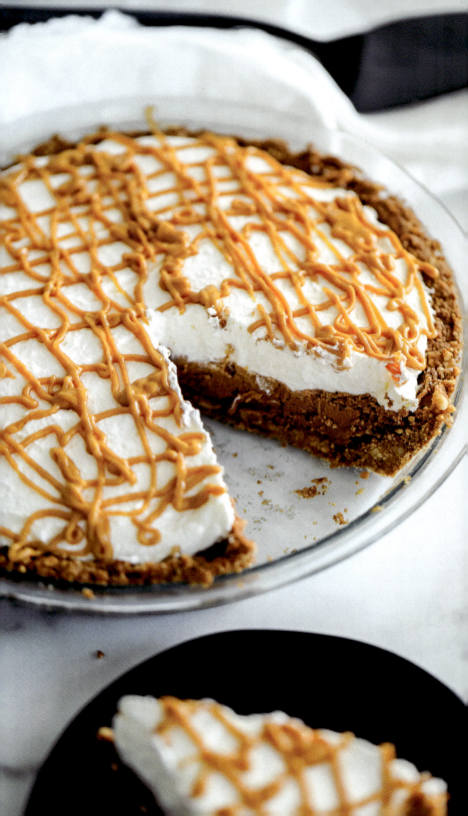

CHOCOLATE PEANUT BUTTER PIE

Makes 12 servings
265 calories / 21.5F / 18C / 5P / per serving

Crust:
2 oz. macadamia nuts
¾ cup Kodiak Cakes Buttermilk Mix
1 Tbs. cocoa powder
¼ cup coconut sugar
¼ cup melted grass-fed butter

Cheesecake:
4 oz. Neufchâtel cream cheese
4 oz. OffBeat Buckeye Brownie Butter
1 serving CSE Brownie Batter
    or Chocolate Peanut Butter Protein Powder
1 cup heavy whipping cream (2 cups whipped)
⅓ cup Swerve confectioners style sweetener

Topping:
1 Tbs. OffBeat Sweet Classic Peanut Butter

1. Preheat the oven to 350 degrees.

2. Add the macadamia nuts to a blender or food processor. Pulse until broken up into a flour. Pour into a bowl and add the Kodiak Cakes, cocoa powder, coconut sugar and melted butter. Mix until well combined. Press into a greased pie tin and bake for 10-12 minutes. Let cool.

3. Place the bowl that you will be using to whip your cream in the freezer for 10 minutes.

4. Add the cream cheese and Buckeye Brownie Butter to a separate bowl and beat for 2-3 minutes or until smooth. Add the protein powder and beat until smooth. Set aside.

5. Remove the bowl from the freezer and add the heavy whipping cream and Swerve sweetener to the bowl. Beat on high for 3-4 minutes or until stiff peaks form. Do not over whip.

6. Beat 1 cup of the whipped cream into the Buckeye Brownie cream cheese mixture. Once combined, spoon the mixture into the pie pan over the crust. Smooth out the top. Spoon the remaining whipped cream on top of the chocolate mixture and smooth out evenly. Drizzle the peanut butter over the top. Let chill in the fridge for 4+ hours or overnight. Slice and serve.

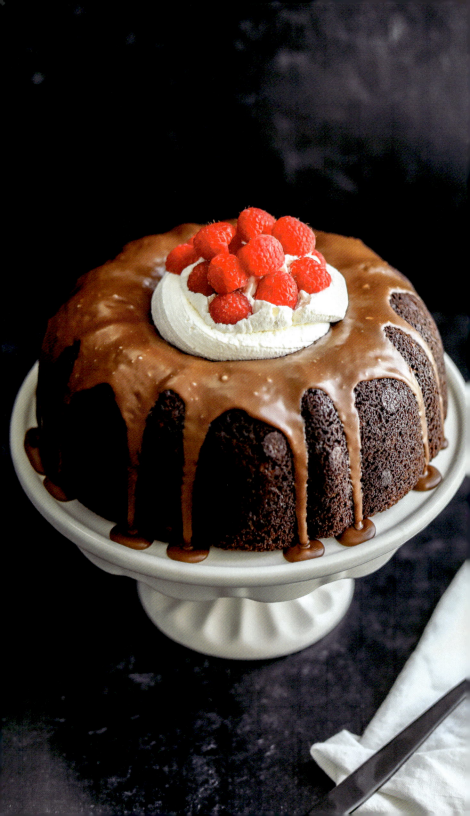

CHOCOLATE ZUCCHINI CAKE

Makes 15 servings
345 calories / 16F / 45C / 5P / per serving

---

2 cups whole wheat pastry flour
¾ cup cocoa powder
2 tsp. baking soda
1 tsp. baking powder
1 tsp. cinnamon
½ tsp. sea salt
1 cup raw honey
¾ cup coconut oil, softened
½ cup coconut sugar
4 large eggs
¾ cup unsweetened applesauce
3 cups grated zucchini
1 cup dark chocolate chips
Optional toppings:
Spray whipped cream
High protein ice cream
Fresh berries

1. Preheat the oven to 350 degrees.

2. Combine the flour, cocoa powder, baking soda, baking powder, cinnamon and salt in a large bowl. Set aside.

3. In a separate bowl beat the honey, coconut oil and coconut sugar together. Beat in the eggs and applesauce. Add to the dry ingredients and mix until just combined. Fold in the grated zucchini and chocolate chips.

4. Pour the batter into a greased 9x13 baking dish or Bundt cake pan. Bake for 40 minutes (might need more time if using a Bundt cake pan). Insert a toothpick into the center of the cake to make sure it is done.

5. Enjoy the cake as is or add toppings of choice. Great with spray whipped cream, high protein ice cream or fresh berries.

*Toppings not included in the macros listed above.

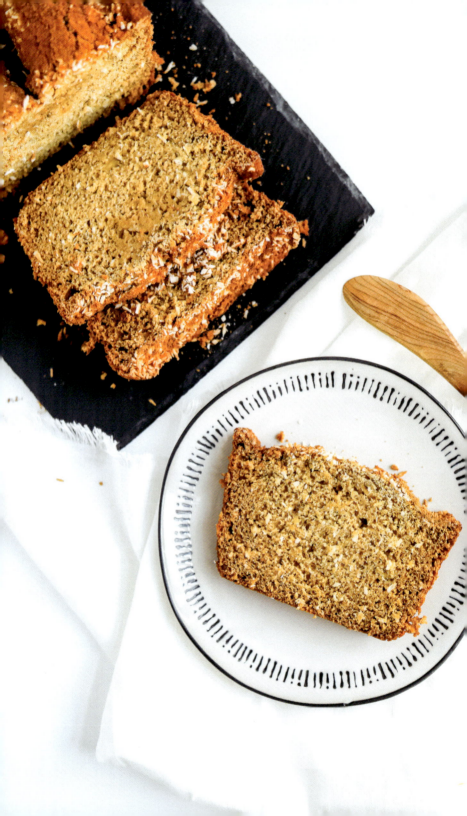

COCONUT BANANA BREAD

Makes 12 servings

175 calories / 5F / 30C / 3P / per serving

2 ripe bananas
3 Tbs. coconut oil
½ cup raw honey
½ cup unsweetened applesauce
1 large egg
1 tsp. vanilla extract
1 ½ cups whole wheat pastry flour
⅓ cup unsweetened shredded coconut
1 tsp. baking soda
½ tsp. baking powder
½ tsp. cinnamon
¼ tsp. sea salt

Toppings:

1 Tbs. coconut sugar
1 Tbs. unsweetened shredded coconut

1. Preheat the oven to 350 degrees.

2. Mash the bananas in a large bowl. Beat in the melted coconut oil, honey and applesauce. Add in the egg and vanilla. Beat on medium speed until well combined.

3. In a separate bowl combine the flour, shredded coconut, baking soda, baking powder, cinnamon and sea salt. Add the dry mixture to the wet mixture. Stir slowly until all the ingredients are just combined.

4. Spray a 9x5 loaf pan with cooking spray and pour the batter into the pan. Sprinkle the coconut sugar and shredded coconut over the top. Bake for 30 minutes, then place a foil tent lightly on top of the bread pan and bake for another 15-20 minutes or until cooked through. Let cool and then slice into 12 servings.

*These also make great, regular sized muffins! Bake at 350 for 20 minutes.

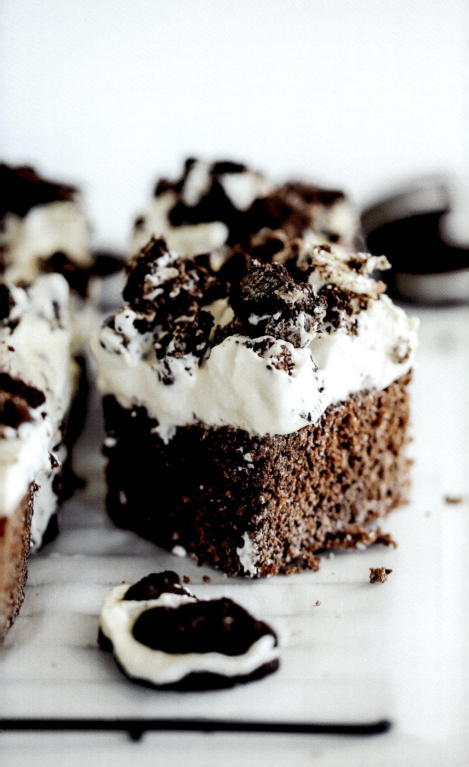

COOKIES & CREAM CAKE
Makes 12 servings
325 calories / 19F / 33.5C / 6.5P / per serving

---

1 ½ cups Kodiak Cakes Dark Chocolate Mix
1 serving CSE Brownie Batter Protein Powder
1 Tbs. black, special dark or regular cocoa powder
½ tsp. baking soda
½ tsp. sea salt
½ cup softened grass-fed butter or melted coconut oil
¾ cup pure maple syrup
4 large eggs
1 tsp. vanilla extract
Toppings:
1 cup heavy whipping cream (2 cups whipped)
2 Tbs. pure maple syrup
½ tsp. vanilla extract
12 Newman-O's Creme Filled Chocolate Cookies
   or other "healthier" creme filled chocolate cookies

1. Preheat oven to 350 degrees. Place the bowl that you will be using to whip your cream in the freezer while you make the cake.

2. Add the Kodiak Cakes Mix, protein powder, cocoa powder, baking soda and sea salt to a bowl. Whisk together until combined; set aside.

3. In a separate bowl add the butter or melted coconut oil and maple syrup. Beat together until smooth. Beat in the eggs and vanilla. Add the dry ingredients to wet ingredients and mix until just combined.

4. Pour batter into a greased 8x8 baking pan. Bake for 25-30 minutes or until cooked through. Let cool.

5. Remove the bowl from the freezer. Add the heavy whipping cream, pure maple syrup and vanilla to the bowl. Beat on high speed for 3-4 minutes or until stiff peaks form. Do not over whip. Spread the whipped cream over the cake and top with crumbled cookies. Store any leftovers in the fridge. Enjoy!

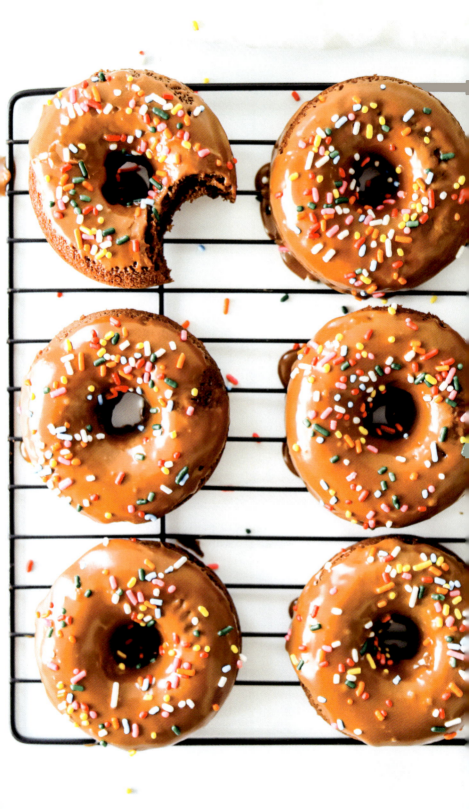

DOUBLE CHOCOLATE CAKE DONUTS

Makes 14 donuts
260 calories / 7.5F / 45.5C / 4.5P / per donut

Donuts:
1 cup whole wheat pastry flour
1 serving CSE Brownie Batter or Chocolate Peanut Butter Protein Powder
½ cup cocoa powder
1 tsp. baking powder
¼ tsp. baking soda
Dash sea salt
¼ cup melted coconut oil
½ cup raw honey
¼ cup pure maple syrup
¼ cup unsweetened applesauce
½ cup cooked, mashed sweet potatoes
½ tsp. vanilla extract
2 large eggs
Frosting:
2 cups powdered sugar
¼ cup pasteurized liquid egg whites
50g chocolate chips
1 tsp. coconut oil
Optional Topping:
Sprinkles

1. Preheat oven to 350 degrees.
2. Add the flour, protein powder, cocoa powder, baking powder, baking soda and sea salt to a bowl. Stir until combined, and set aside.
3. In a separate bowl, add the melted coconut oil, honey, maple syrup, applesauce and mashed sweet potatoes. Beat until well combined. Add the vanilla and eggs. Mix. Add the dry mixture to the wet and mix until just combined.
4. Grease a donut pan. Pour the mixture into a large Ziploc bag. Cut one of the corners off the bag about ½ inch wide. Pipe the batter into the donut molds, filling about ¾ of the way full. Bake for 12-15 minutes. Let cool for a few minutes, then remove from pan and transfer each donut to a cooling rack.
5. Add the chocolate chips and coconut oil to a small bowl. Melt in the microwave for 1-2 minutes, stirring every 30 seconds.
6. Add the powdered sugar and egg whites to a mixing bowl and beat until well combined. Add the melted chocolate chip mixture and beat until combined.
7. Dip the top of each donut into the frosting and return to the cooling rack. Top immediately with sprinkles and let the frosting harden. Store leftovers in the fridge.

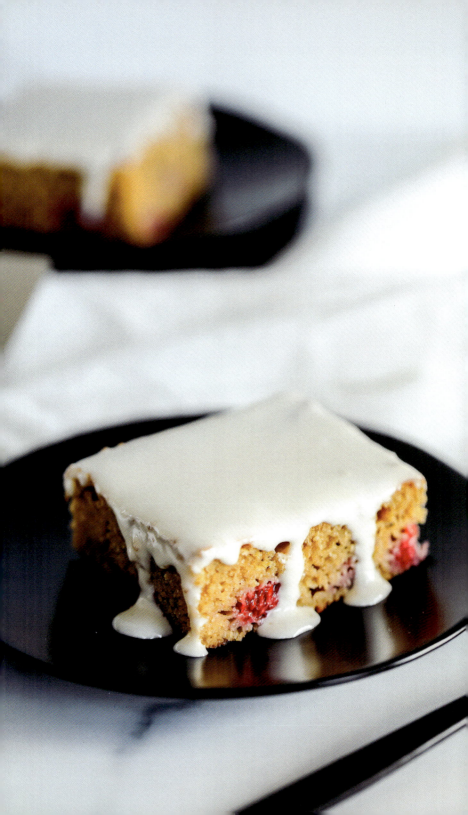

LEMON RASPBERRY BREAKFAST CAKE

Makes 20 servings
240 calories / 12F / 29.5C / 5.5P / per serving

1 cup grass-fed butter
1 cup xylitol natural sweetener
¾ cup coconut sugar
4 large eggs
1 cup nonfat, vanilla Greek yogurt
2 lemons, zest of
2 ¼ cups Kodiak Cakes Buttermilk Mix
½ tsp. sea salt
½ tsp. baking powder
½ tsp. baking soda
1 cup fresh raspberries
¼ cup Kodiak Cakes Buttermilk Mix
Cake Glaze:
1 cup powdered sugar
2 Tbs. melted, grass-fed butter
2 Tbs. pasteurized liquid egg whites
½ tsp. almond extract

1. Preheat the oven to 350 degrees.

2. Beat the butter, xylitol and coconut sugar together in a large bowl. Add in one egg at a time and mix until well-combined. In a separate bowl, mix the Greek yogurt together with the lemon zest, then fold into the sugar mixture. Set aside.

3. Add 2 ¼ cups Kodiak Cakes Mix, sea salt, baking powder and baking soda to a separate bowl. Stir until combined. Add the dry ingredients to the wet ingredients and mix until just combined. Toss the raspberries in ¼ cup Kodiak Cakes Mix, then fold the fresh raspberries into the batter.

4. Pour the batter evenly into a greased 9x13 baking dish. Bake for 35-40 minutes or until the top is golden and the cake is cooked through. Let cool.

5. Once the cake has cooled completely, add all of the icing ingredients together in a bowl and beat until smooth. Drizzle the icing evenly over the cake. Enjoy!

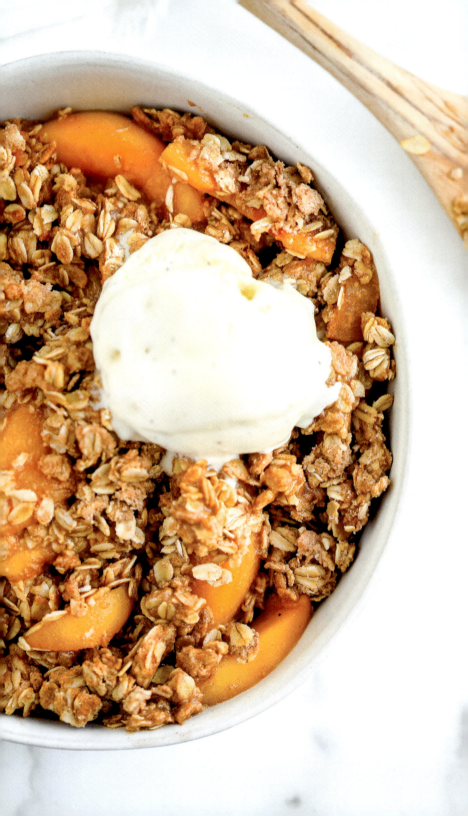

PEACH CRISP

Makes 12 servings
235 calories / 7F / 39C / 6P / per serving

2 lbs. ripe peaches, peeled, pitted and sliced
¼ cup coconut sugar
1 Tbs. lemon juice
½ tsp. almond extract
Crumble Topping:
2 cups old-fashioned rolled oats
1 ½ cups Cinnamon Oat Kodiak Cakes Mix
½ cup raw honey
1 Tbs. cinnamon
¼ tsp. sea salt
6 Tbs. grass-fed butter or coconut oil, chopped
Optional toppings:
Spray whipped cream
High protein ice cream

1. Preheat the oven to 375 degrees.

2. In a large bowl, add the peaches, coconut sugar, lemon juice and almond extract. Mix until the peaches are well coated. Pour into a greased 9x13 glass baking dish.

3. Combine all the topping ingredients together in a bowl with hands or a pastry cutter until thick and crumbly. Press on top of the peach mixture.

4. Bake for 20-25 minutes. Serve warm. Top each individual serving with spray whipped cream or high protein ice cream. Enjoy!

*Toppings not included in macros listed above.

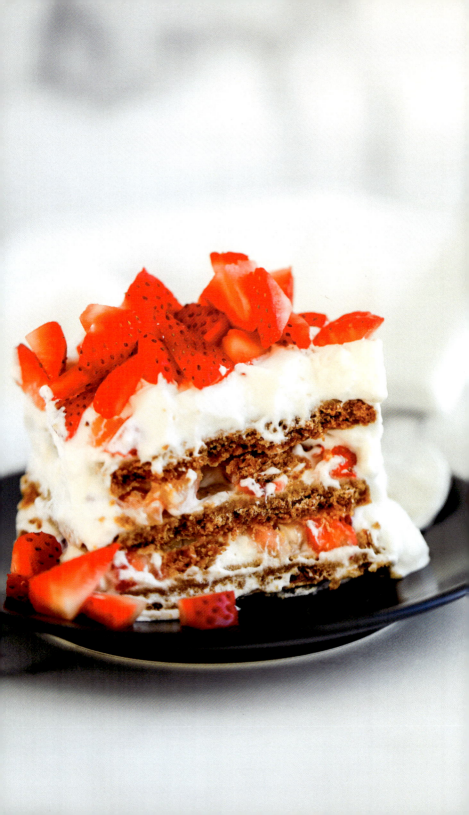

STRAWBERRIES & CREAM ICEBOX CAKE

Makes 12 servings
300 calories / 21F / 26C / 1.5P / per serving

---

12 Homemade Graham Cookies (recipe on page 133)
2 cups heavy whipping cream
¼ cup pure maple syrup or raw honey
1 tsp. vanilla extract
4 cups of strawberries

1. Place the bowl that you will be using to whip your cream in the freezer while you make the Homemade Graham Cookies.

2. Make the Homemade Graham Cookies. Let cool completely.

3. Wash and slice the strawberries. Store in the fridge until ready to use.

4. Remove the bowl from the freezer. Add the heavy whipping cream, sweetener and vanilla to the chilled bowl. Beat on high speed for 3-4 minutes or until stiff peaks start to form. Don't over whip.

5. Layer in a 8x8 baking pan: a thin layer of the whipping cream on the bottom, 4 Homemade Grahams, ⅓ of the whipping cream and ⅓ of the strawberries. Repeat layers 2 more times. Store in the fridge 6+ hours or overnight. Slice and serve!

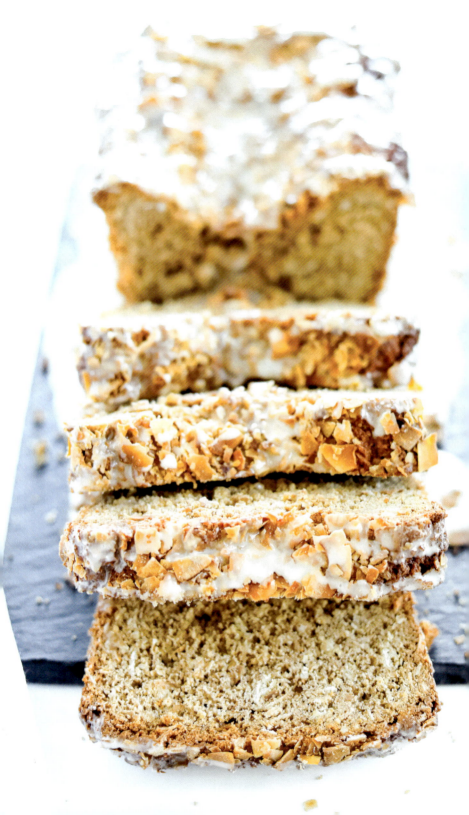

TOASTED COCONUT POUND CAKE
Makes 12 servings
310 calories / 13F / 40C / 9P / per serving

Coconut Cake:
¾ cup coconut butter
¾ cup xylitol natural sweetener
¼ cup coconut sugar
¼ cup unsweetened applesauce
1 tsp. coconut extract
4 large eggs
1 ½ cups Kodiak Cakes Cinnamon Oat Mix
½ cup unsweetened flaked coconut, divided
1 tsp. baking powder
½ tsp. baking soda
½ tsp. sea salt
Coconut Glaze:
1 cup powdered sugar
3 Tbs. pasteurized liquid egg whites
1 tsp. coconut extract

1. Preheat the oven to 325 degrees. Spray a 9x5 loaf pan with cooking spray.

2. Add the coconut butter, xylitol and coconut sugar to a large bowl and beat until combined. Mix in the applesauce and coconut extract. Beat eggs, one at a time, into the batter until smooth.

3. In a separate bowl whisk together the Kodiak Cakes mix, ¼ cup flaked coconut, baking powder, baking soda and sea salt. Fold the dry ingredients into the wet ingredients and stir until just combined.

4. Pour the batter into the greased loaf pan and spread the batter out evenly. Top with the remaining ¼ cup of flaked coconut. Bake for 60-65 minutes total. Foil tent the cake after about 35-40 minutes of baking, so the top doesn't burn. When done, insert a toothpick into the center of the cake to check if your cake is done. Let cool for 30-60 minutes in the pan.

5. In a small bowl, whisk together the powdered sugar, egg whites and coconut extract. Using a toothpick, poke holes all over the top of the cake. Drizzle the Coconut Glaze over the pound cake and let it seep down through the holes. Let the glaze harden and enjoy.

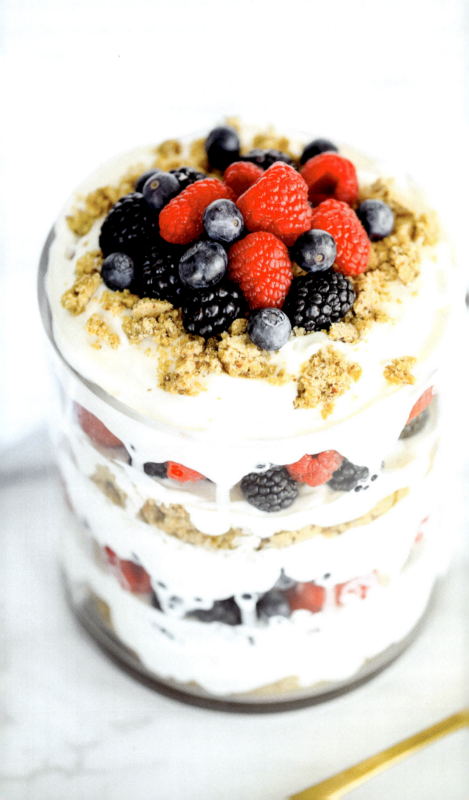

TRIPLE BERRY CREAM CHEESE TRIFLE

Makes 16 servings
225 calories / 14F / 20C / 6P / per serving

Crust:

¼ cup melted coconut oil or grass-fed butter
⅓ cup coconut sugar
1 large egg
½ tsp. vanilla extract
2 Tbs. unsweetened applesauce
2 Tbs. flaxseed meal
2 Tbs. cold water
2 cups oat flour
½ cup almond flour
¼ tsp. sea salt

Coconut Cream Cheese Filling:

1 cup canned coconut cream
2 Tbs. pure maple syrup
8 oz. Neufchâtel cream cheese
1 cup nonfat, plain Greek yogurt
2 droppers full vanilla stevia drops
½ tsp. vanilla extract

Toppings:

1 ½ cups sliced strawberries
1 ½ cups blueberries
1 ½ cups blackberries

1. Preheat the oven to 350 degrees. Place the bowl that you will be using to whip your coconut cream in the freezer.

2. Beat the butter or coconut oil and coconut sugar together in a large bowl. Add the egg, vanilla, applesauce, flaxseed meal and water. Mix until well combined. Add in the oat flour, almond flour and sea salt; mix well. Press evenly into a greased 9x13 baking dish. Bake for 20 minutes. It should look golden and lightly browned on the edges. Remove and let cool in the pan. Once cool, cut into 16 squares and let chill in the fridge for one hour.

3. Beat the cream cheese together with the vanilla stevia drops and vanilla extract until smooth. Slowly beat in the Greek yogurt until smooth; set aside.

4. Remove the bowl from the freezer and add the coconut cream and pure maple syrup. Beat on high speed for 4-5 minutes or until stiff peaks form. Fold in the cream cheese mixture. Store in the fridge for 1 hour.

5. Add 8 of the cookie squares to the bottom of a greased 9x13 pan and then layer ½ of the whipped cream cheese mixture and ½ of the berries. Repeat the layers and store in the fridge until ready to serve.

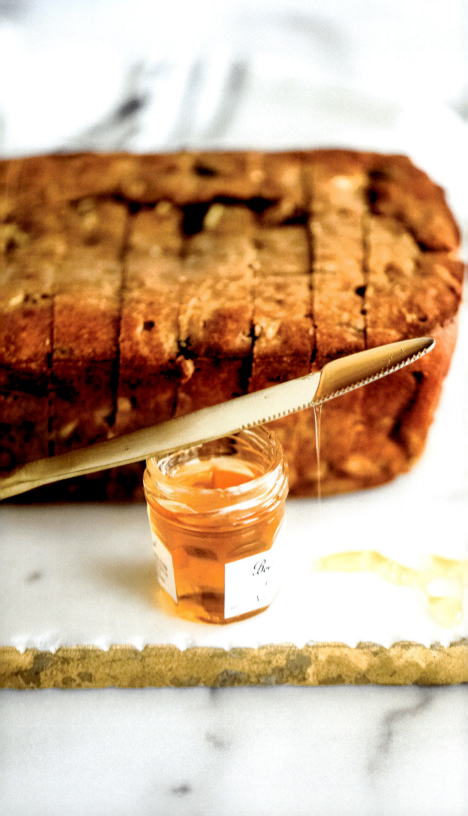

ZUCCHINI BANANA BREAD

Makes 12 servings
160 calories / 3.5F / 30C / 4P / per serving

1 cup grated zucchini
1 ripe mashed banana
2 Tbs. melted coconut oil
1 cup coconut sugar
½ cup unsweetened applesauce
2 large eggs
1 tsp. vanilla extract
1 ¼ cups whole wheat pastry flour
1 serving CSE Simply Vanilla Protein Powder
½ Tbs. cinnamon
¾ tsp. baking soda
¾ tsp. baking powder
½ tsp. sea salt

1. Preheat the oven to 350 degrees.

2. Grate the zucchini and mash the banana.

3. Add the mashed banana, zucchini, melted coconut oil, coconut sugar, applesauce, eggs and vanilla to a large bowl. Whisk until well combined.

4. In a separate bowl add the pastry flour, protein powder, cinnamon, baking soda, baking powder and sea salt. Whisk until combined. Add the dry ingredients to the wet ingredients and mix until just combined.

5. Grease a 9x5 glass loaf pan or a muffin tin. Pour the batter into the loaf pan or muffin tin. Fill each muffin ¾ of the way full; should make 12 muffins.

6. For a bread loaf, bake 50-55 minutes; for muffins bake 20-25 minutes. Let cool 5-10 minutes in the pan and then transfer to a cooling rack. Slice and enjoy as is or top with raw honey. Store the leftovers in the fridge.

FROZEN TREATS

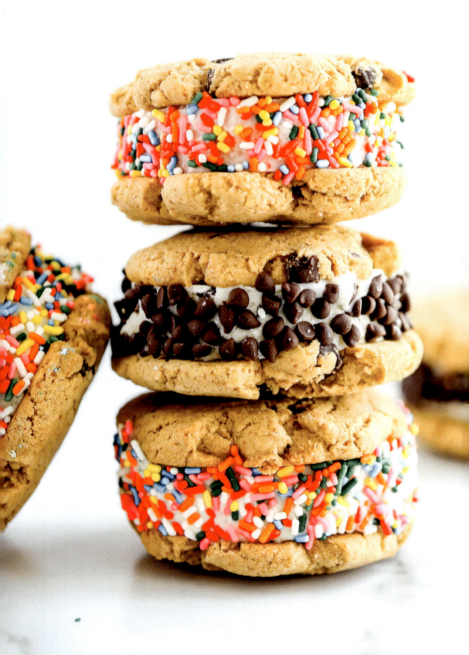

I'LL STOP THE WORLD AND MELT WITH YOU

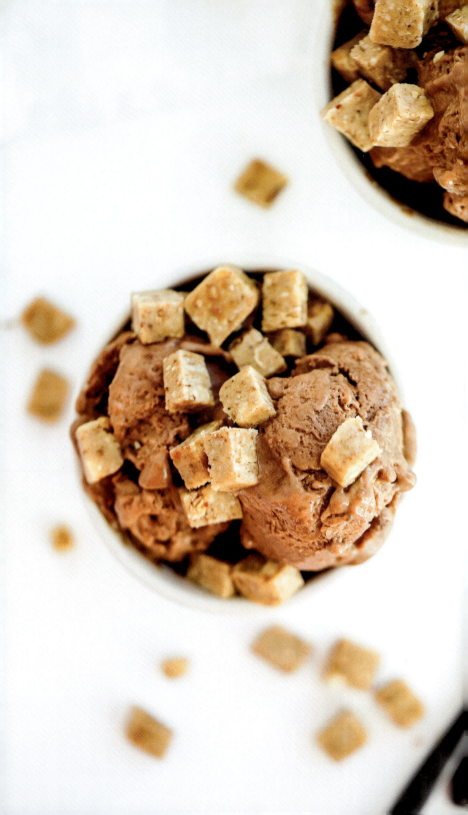

CHOCO-BANANA NICE CREAM

Makes 4 servings
220 calories / 5.5F / 23.5C / 18P / per serving

200g frozen banana slices
2 Tbs. unsweetened almond milk
1 Tbs. OffBeat Butter of choice or
    natural almond butter/peanut butter
1 tsp. vanilla extract
Vanilla stevia drops, optional for sweetness
¼ tsp. xanthan gum, optional for thickness
2 ½ servings (85g) CSE Brownie Batter
    or Chocolate Peanut Butter Protein Powder
Pinch sea salt
Topping:
1 G2G Protein Bar, chopped

1. Place the frozen bananas, almond milk, nut butter, vanilla, stevia and xanthan gum in a high-powered blender. Pulse until the bananas are broken up. Add in the protein powder and pinch of sea salt and blend until smooth. Enjoy as is or place in the freezer for 2+ hours for a thicker consistency.

2. Scoop ¼ of the Choco-Banana Nice Cream into a bowl and top with ¼ of the chopped protein bar.

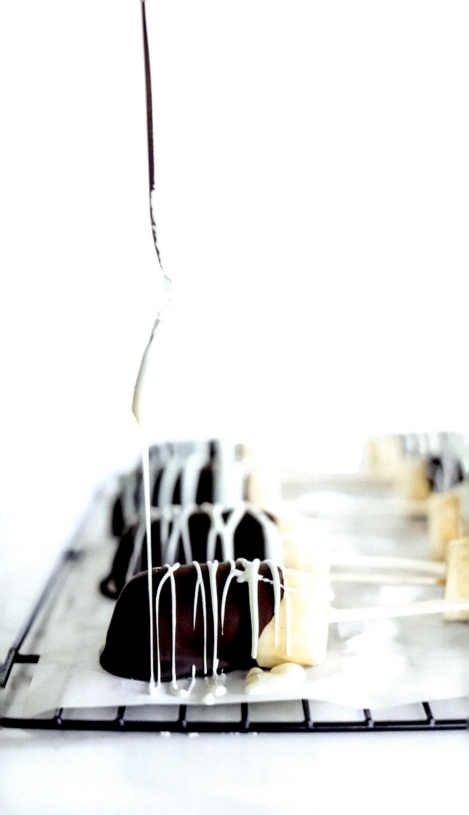

CHOCOLATE ALOHA DIPPED BANANAS

Makes 8 servings
250 calories / 14F / 30C / 3P / per serving

4 (120g each) bananas
½ cup OffBeat Aloha Butter
   or natural almond/peanut butter
½ cup dark chocolate chips
¼ cup white chocolate chips

1. Slice each banana in half. Slice off the pointed edge of each half banana. Press a popsicle stick into the end of each one, about ¾ of the way through. Place on a baking sheet lined with parchment paper. Freeze 2+ hours.

2. Stir the Aloha Butter, then pour it into a cup. Dip each frozen banana into the butter, leaving a little bit of the banana exposed. Let the excess drip off, then place back onto the baking sheet. Return the baking sheet to the freezer until ready to dip into the chocolate.

3. Add the dark chocolate chips to a tall cup. Microwave for 30 seconds at a time, stirring in between, until completely melted and smooth. Should take about 60-90 seconds total.

4. Dip each banana into the melted chocolate. Let the excess drip off, then place back onto the baking sheet.

5. Melt the white chocolate chips in a small bowl in the microwave. Drizzle over the double dipped bananas.

6. Return all the dipped bananas to the freezer. Let the chocolate harden and enjoy!

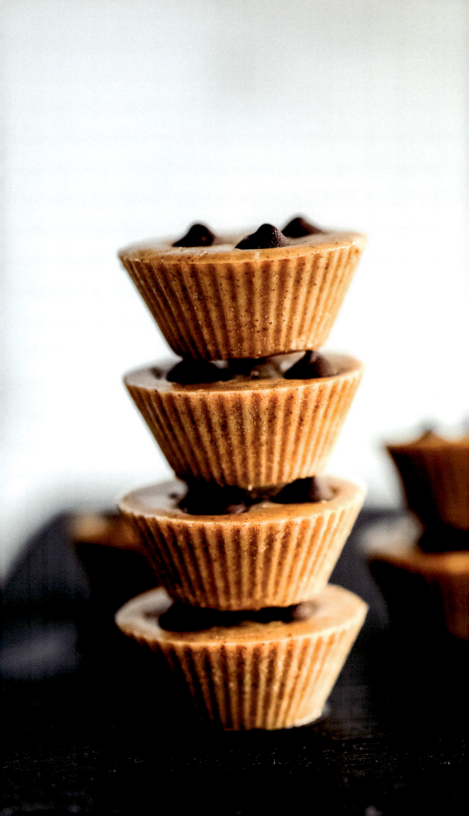

DARK CHOCOLATE SEA SALT CARAMEL FUDGE

Makes 16 servings
115 calories / 9.5F / 7C / 2.5P / per serving

---

1 cup OffBeat Salted Caramel Butter
   or natural almond butter
2 Tbs. coconut oil
2 Tbs. pure maple syrup
2 Tbs. dark chocolate chips

1. Add the Salted Caramel Butter, coconut oil, pure maple syrup and chocolate chips to a small saucepan. Melt down over low/medium heat. Stir constantly until smooth and pourable.

2. Place 16 mini silicone muffin liners on a baking sheet. Pour the chocolate caramel mixture into each one, filling almost to the top.

3. Freeze 4+ hours or overnight. Let thaw on the counter for 5-10 minutes before enjoying.

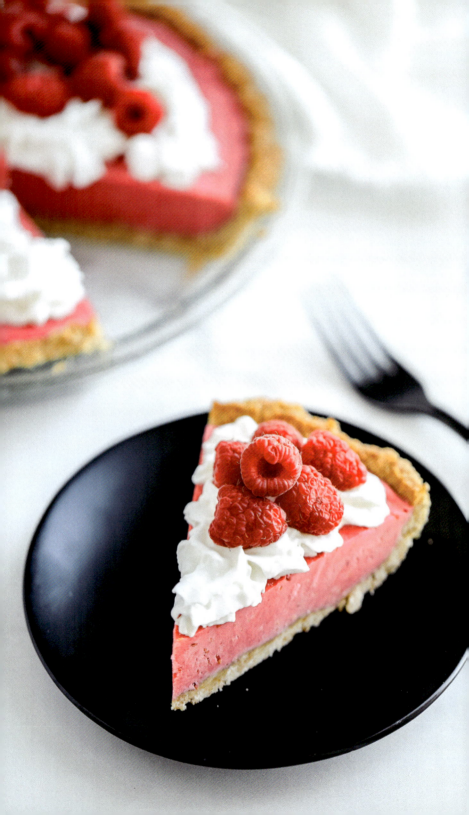

FROZEN RASPBERRY SORBET PIE

Makes 8 servings
300 calories / 15F / 21.5C / 4.5P / per serving

Pie crust:
¼ cup OffBeat Lemon Coconut Bliss Butter
   or natural coconut butter
¼ cup melted grass-fed butter
¼ cup coconut sugar
½ serving (16g) CSE Simply Vanilla Protein Powder
2 Tbs. flaxseed meal
1 cup almond flour
½ tsp. vanilla extract
¼ tsp. sea salt

Pie filling:
1 cup canned coconut cream
2 Tbs. pure maple syrup
2 cups fresh raspberries
¼ cup xylitol natural sweetener
½ Tbs. fresh lemon juice

Toppings per serving:
2 Tbs. spray whipped cream
6 fresh raspberries

1. Preheat the oven to 400 degrees.

2. Add the nut butter, melted butter, coconut sugar, protein powder, flaxseed meal, almond flour, vanilla extract and sea salt to a large bowl. Mix until well combined.

3. Press the crust dough into the bottom and up the sides of a greased pie pan. Bake for 8-10 minutes. Remove from the oven and let cool completely.

4. Add the coconut cream, pure maple syrup, raspberries, xylitol and lemon juice to a blender. Blend until smooth. Pour the mixture into the pie pan over the crust. Smooth out the top and freeze until firm. Let thaw about 10-20 minutes before eating. Top each individual serving with whipped cream and fresh raspberries. Enjoy!

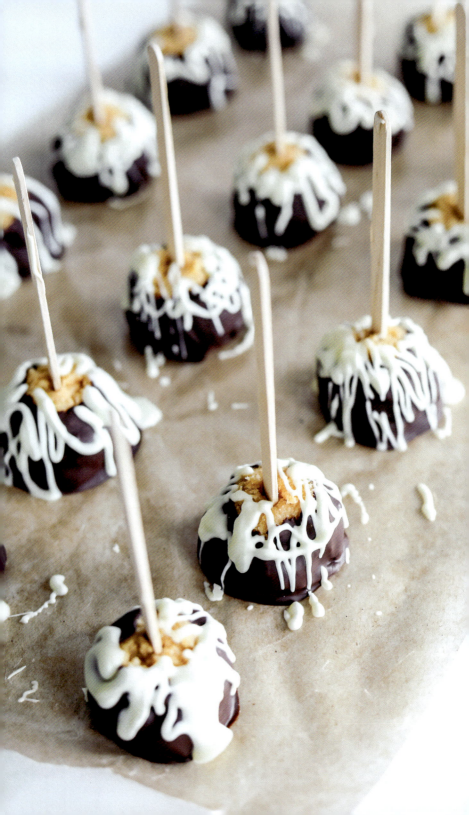

FROZEN TRUFFLE POPS

Makes 24 servings
165 calories / 12.5F / 9C / 4P / per serving

4 oz. Neufchâtel cream cheese
½ cup grass-fed butter
1 cup OffBeat Sweet Classic Peanut Butter
2 Tbs. xylitol natural sweetener
½ cup CSE Simply Vanilla Protein Powder
Toppings:
¾ cup dark chocolate chips
¼ cup white chocolate chips
2 tsp. coconut oil

1. Add the cream cheese, butter and peanut butter to a mixing bowl. Beat together until smooth. Add in the xylitol and protein powder. Mix until well combined and fluffy. Cover and place in the freezer for 30 minutes or until firm.

2. Using a small cookie scoop, scoop into balls and place on a baking sheet lined with parchment paper. Stick a popsicle stick into the top of each one. Freeze for another 30 minutes.

3. Add the chocolate chips and the white chocolate chips to two separate bowls with 1 tsp. coconut oil in each. Melt in the micro-wave for 30 seconds at a time, stirring in between until completely melted and smooth. Usually takes about 60-90 seconds total.

4. Dip each peanut butter pop into the dark chocolate dip and place back on the parchment paper. Drizzle the white chocolate over the top. Return to the freezer until ready to eat. Enjoy!

*Try swapping in a different flavor of OffBeat Butter or CSE protein powder for a fun spin on the recipe.

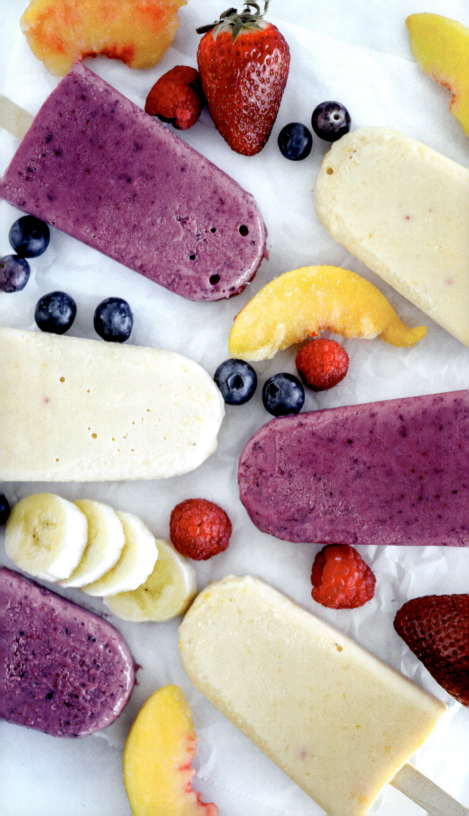

FRUIT & YOGURT POPS
Makes 8 popsicles
75 calories / 1.5F / 13C / 3P / per popsicle

---

2 cups ripe fruit of choice
  (peaches, berries, mangos, bananas, pineapple)
1 cup full-fat plain Greek yogurt
½ Tbs. lemon juice
¼ cup raw honey
½ tsp. vanilla extract
  (or other extract of choice: coconut, almond, banana)

1. Preheat oven to 350 degrees.

2. Spread the fruit onto a baking sheet lined with parchment paper. Roast in the oven for about 30 minutes.

3. Add the fruit to a blender with the yogurt, lemon juice, honey and extract of choice. Blend until smooth.

4. Pour the fruity yogurt mixture into popsicle molds and stick a popsicle stick into the top of each one. Freeze 6+ hours or over-night.

5. Let thaw about 5-10 minutes before removing from the popsicle molds. Enjoy!!

*macros will differ slightly depending on which fruit you use.

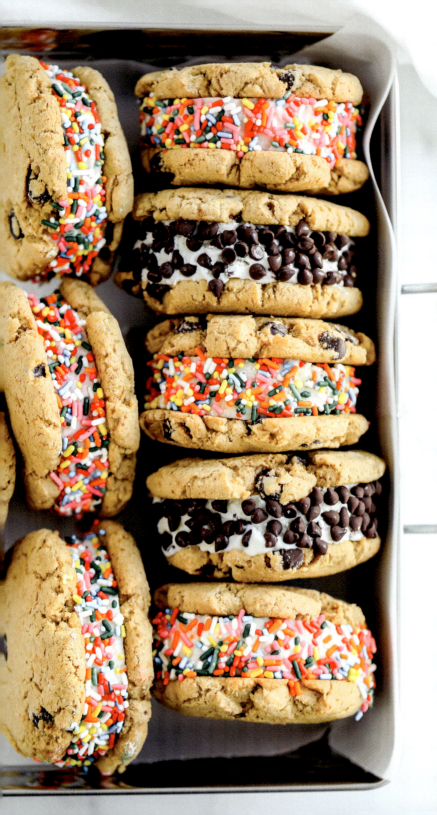

ICE CREAM COOKIE SANDWICHES
Makes 18 cookies / 9 cookie sandwiches
280 calories / 14.5F / 39C / 7P / per ½ of a cookie sandwich

1 cup grass-fed butter
¾ cup brown sugar or coconut sugar
½ cup sugar in the raw
   or xylitol natural sweetener
2 large eggs
1 Tbs. vanilla extract
2 ½ cups whole wheat flour
1 tsp. baking soda
½ tsp. sea salt
½ cup dark chocolate chips
3 pints of high protein ice cream, any flavor
Optional toppings:
Sprinkles
Mini chocolate chips
Chopped nuts

1. Preheat the oven to 375 degrees.

2. Add the butter, brown sugar and sugar in the raw to a mixing bowl. Mix them on medium speed until creamed together and smooth. Add the eggs and vanilla. Mix until combined.

3. Add the whole wheat flour, baking soda and salt to a separate bowl. Whisk until combined. Add the dry ingredients to the wet ingredients and mix until just combined. Fold in the chocolate chips.

4. Using a large cookie scoop, scoop the cookie dough onto a baking sheet lined with parchment paper. Flatten each cookie with the bottom of a greased cup. Bake for 8-10 minutes. Let cool on the baking sheet for 2 minutes, then transfer to a cooling rack. Once completely cooled, place in a large Ziploc bag and freeze for 2+ hours.

5. Remove the lid from the ice cream and then cut off the bottom of the carton with a sharp knife. Dump the ice cream out of the carton onto a cutting board, trying to keep the shape intact. Slice each pint of ice cream into 3 rounds. Sandwich each round, pressing firmly, between two cookies.

6. Pour the toppings of choice into a bowl. Using a spoon, scoop the toppings up out of the bowl and sprinkle over the ice cream in between the cookies. Use the back side of the spoon to press the toppings into the ice cream. Return to the freezer until ready to eat.
*Optional toppings not included in the macros listed above.

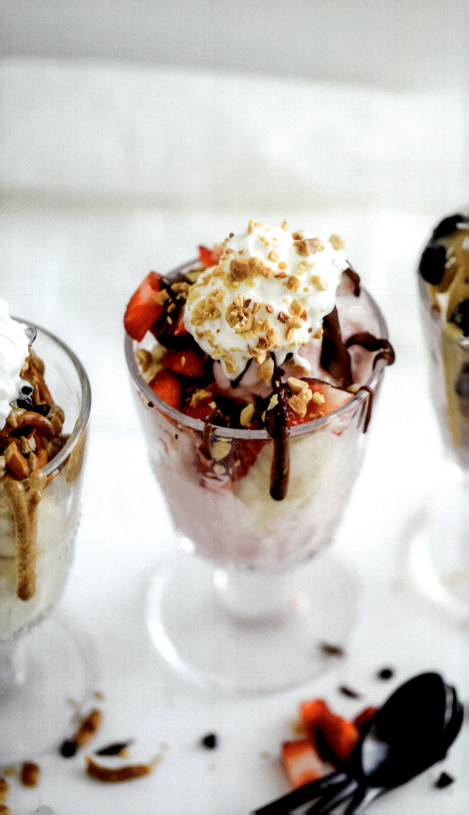

CARAMEL PRETZEL CHOCOLATE CHIP SUNDAE
Makes 1 serving
360 calories / 10F / 56C / 13P

¾ of a banana, sliced
1 cup Vanilla Bean Halo Top Ice Cream
½ Tbs. OffBeat Salted Caramel Butter
2 Tbs. chopped pretzels
1 tsp. mini chocolate chips
2 Tbs. spray whipped cream

STRAWBERRY BUCKEYE BROWNIE SUNDAE
Makes 1 serving
315 calories / 11F / 43C / 13P

¾ of a banana, sliced
1 cup Strawberry Halo Top Ice Cream
½ Tbs. OffBeat Buckeye Brownie Butter
2 Tbs. chopped strawberries
½ Tbs. chopped peanuts
2 Tbs. spray whipped cream

CHOCOLATE PEANUT BUTTER SUNDAE
Makes 1 serving
320 calories / 12F / 53C / 12.5P

¾ of a banana, sliced
1 cup Chocolate Halo Top Ice Cream
½ Tbs. OffBeat Sweet Classic Peanut Butter
1 Tbs. mini chocolate chips
2 Tbs. spray whipped cream

BLUEBERRY COCONUT SUNDAE
Makes 1 serving
350 calories / 11.5F / 59.5C / 12P

¾ of a banana, sliced
1 cup Blueberry Crumble Halo Top Ice Cream
½ Tbs. OffBeat Lemon Coconut Bliss Butter
2 Tbs. fresh blueberries
½ Tbs. unsweetened shredded coconut
2 Tbs. spray whipped cream

1. Add the sliced bananas to the bottom of a bowl or cup. Scoop the ice cream on top of the bananas, then drizzle with OffBeat Butter. Sprinkle all the other toppings over the ice cream. Enjoy with a spoon!

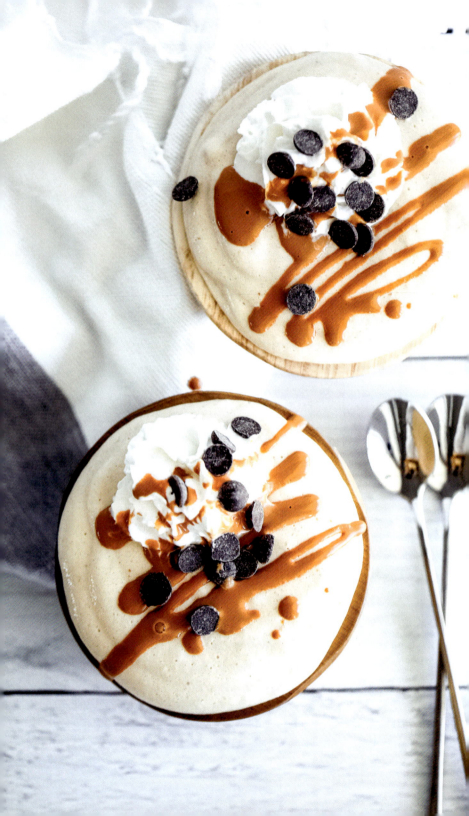

PB LOVER'S ICE CREAM

Makes 2 servings
230 calories / 5F / 27.5C / 19P / per serving

½ cup low-fat cottage cheese
2 Tbs. unsweetened almond milk
¼ cup powdered peanut butter
½ serving (16g) CSE Simply Vanilla, Chocolate Peanut Butter,
   or Brownie Batter Protein Powder
Vanilla stevia drops, optional
½ cup unsweetened almond milk
150g frozen banana slices
¼ tsp. xanthan gum, optional to thicken
8-10 (130g) ice cubes
8g mini chocolate chips

1. Add the cottage cheese, 2 Tbs. almond milk, powdered peanut butter, protein powder and stevia drops to a blender. Blend until smooth. Mixture should be thick.

2. Pour into an ice cube tray and freeze 4+ hours or overnight.

3. Add the ½ cup almond milk, the frozen cubes, frozen banana slices and ice to a high-powered blender. Blend until smooth. Pour into two bowls.

4. Top each serving with 4g mini chocolate chips. Enjoy!

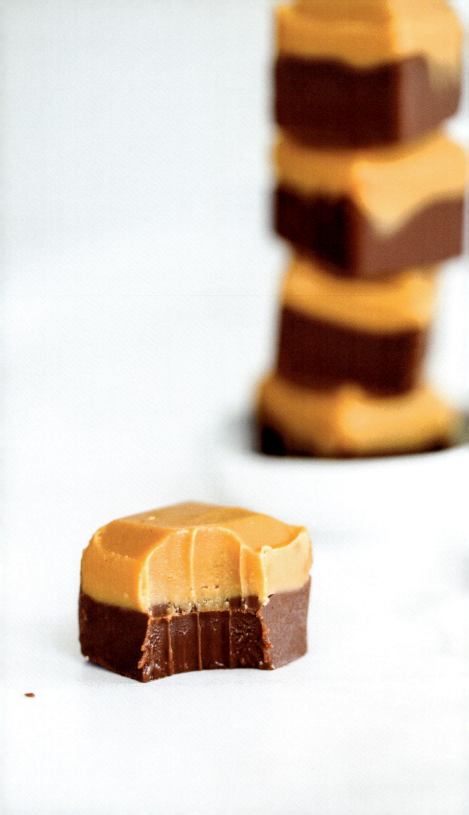

PEANUT BUTTER CUP FREEZER FUDGE

Makes 6 servings
155 calories / 12.5F / 6C / 5P / per serving

¼ cup OffBeat Sweet Classic Peanut Butter
   or natural peanut butter
1 Tbs. pure maple syrup
¼ tsp. vanilla extract
¼ cup OffBeat Buckeye Brownie Peanut Butter
   or natural peanut butter
1 Tbs. grass-fed butter or coconut oil

1. Mix the Sweet Classic PB with the maple syrup and vanilla. Spoon ½ Tbs. of the mixture into an ice cube tray, making 6 servings. Freeze for 30+ minutes.

2. Add the Buckeye Brownie Peanut Butter and the coconut oil into a bowl. Microwave for 10-20 seconds or until the butter/coconut oil is melted. Whisk together until smooth. Spoon ½ Tbs. of the chocolate mixture on top of the peanut butter mixture in the ice cube tray. Freeze 4+ hours. Enjoy!

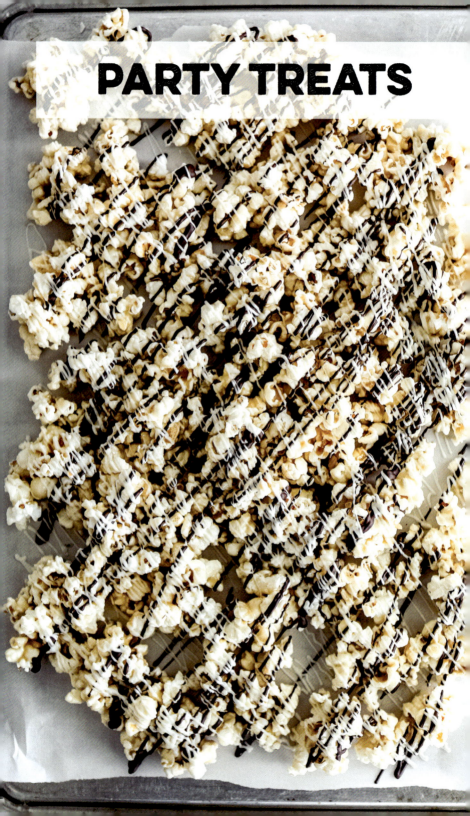

PARTY TREATS

FOOD.
FRIENDS.
SUNSHINE.

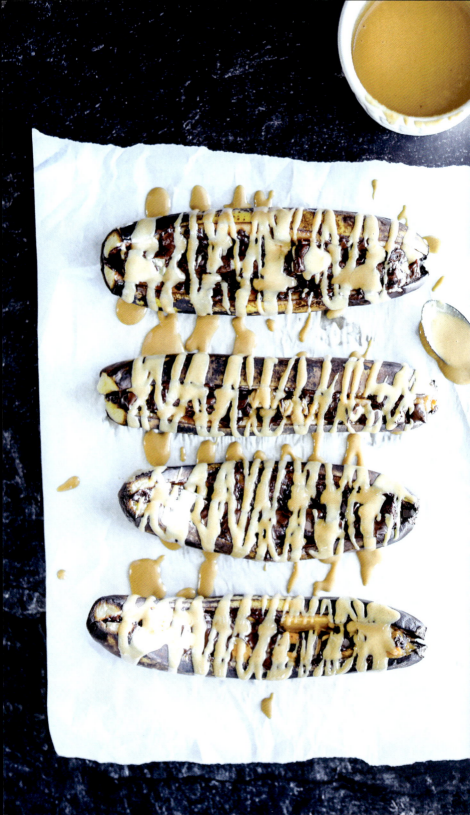

CAMPFIRE BANANA BOAT

Makes 1 serving
350 calories / 15F / 50C / 11.5P

---

1 banana
1 Tbs. dark chocolate chips
½ of a protein bar (we like G2G or GoMacro best in this recipe)
½ Tbs. OffBeat Sweet Classic Peanut Butter
   or natural peanut butter

1. Coarsely chop the protein bar and slice the banana down the middle, lengthwise, keeping the peel on. Sprinkle the chopped protein bar and chocolate chips into the center of each banana.

2. Set the banana in the center of a piece of foil and wrap up tight. Place the bananas in the hot coals of a campfire for 5-10 minutes. Open up the foil and drizzle the peanut butter over the top of the banana. Enjoy warm with a spoon!

*You can also bake these in the oven at 400 degrees for 10 minutes.

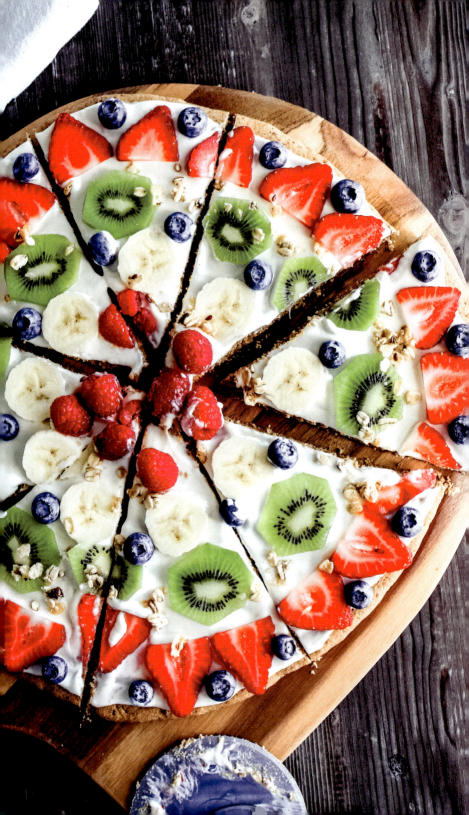

FRUIT PIZZA

Makes 16 servings
205 calories / 8.5F / 28C / 4.5P / per serving

Cookie Crust:
½ cup grass-fed butter
¾ cup organic coconut sugar
1 large egg
1 ½ Tbs. cold water
1 tsp. vanilla extract
2 cups whole wheat pastry flour
¼ tsp. sea salt
¼ tsp. baking soda

Frosting:
¾ cup whipped cream cheese
1 Tbs. raw honey
½ Tbs. almond milk
½ tsp. vanilla extract
½ serving (16g) CSE Simply Vanilla Protein Powder

Toppings:
1 peeled and sliced kiwi
½ cup sliced strawberries
¼ of a banana, sliced
¼ cup blueberries
¼ cup raspberries

1. Preheat the oven to 375 degrees.

2. Beat the butter and sugar together in a bowl. Once smooth add in the egg, water and vanilla extract. In a separate bowl, combine the flour, salt and baking soda. Add the wet ingredients to the dry and mix well.

3. Place the dough on a large piece of parchment paper and roll out into a giant circle about ⅛ inch thick. Flour the surface of the dough or the rolling pin, if needed. Place the parchment paper and cookie dough onto a large baking sheet. Bake for 8-10 minutes or until lightly brown on the edges. Let cool completely.

4. For the frosting, add the cream cheese, honey, almond milk and vanilla extract to a bowl; mix until smooth. Slowly beat in the protein powder until well incorporated. Do not over mix.

5. Spread the frosting evenly on top of the cookie. Decorate the cookie with all the fruit toppings. Slice into 16 servings and enjoy cold.

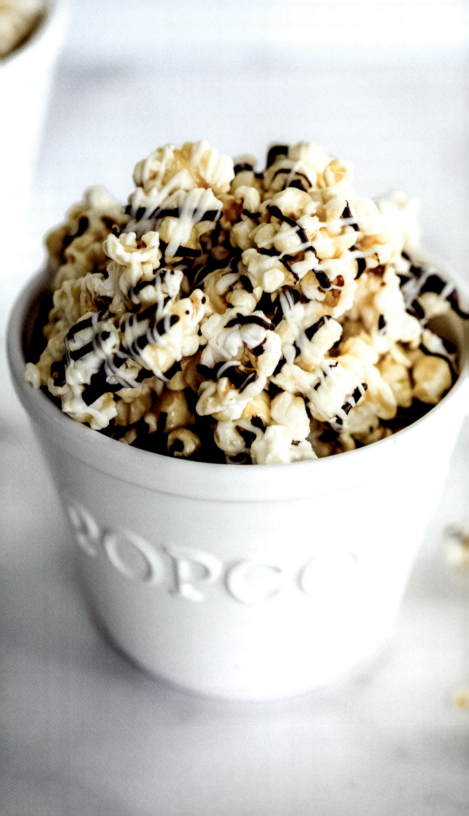

SALTED CARAMEL CORN

Makes 8 servings
265 calories / 11F / 38C / 4P / per serving

12 cups air-popped popcorn
½ cup OffBeat Salted Caramel Butter
  or natural almond butter
½ cup raw honey
1 tsp. vanilla or caramel extract
¼ cup dark chocolate chips
¼ cup white chocolate chips
Dash sea salt

1. Add the Salted Caramel Butter, honey and vanilla to a sauce pan and heat on low. Stir constantly until melted together and smooth.

2. Place the popcorn in a large bowl. Pour the mixture over the top and stir until well coated. Dump onto a large baking sheet lined with parchment paper.

3. Place the chocolate chips in two separate bowls. Melt the chocolate chips in the microwave for 30 seconds at a time, stirring in between until smooth.

4. Pour each flavor of chocolate into a separate ziploc bag and cut a small hole in the corner. Drizzle over the popcorn and then sprinkle sea salt over the top. Let the chocolate harden, then dig in.

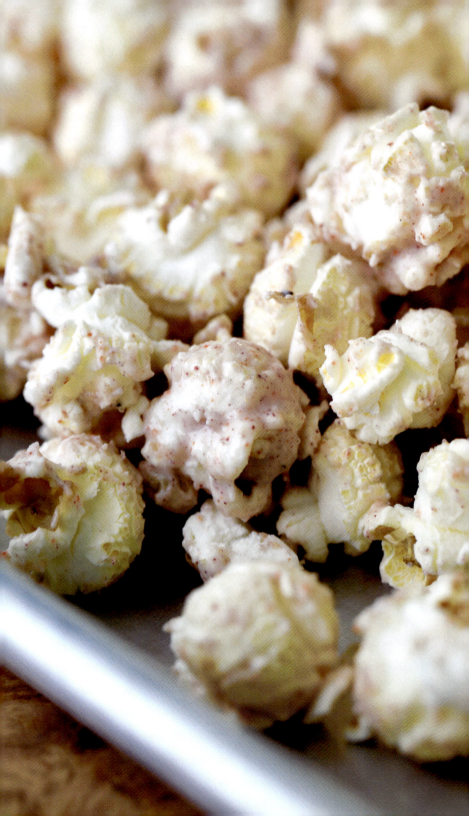

SUPER BERRY WHITE CHOCOLATE POPCORN

Makes 4 servings
115 calories / 6.5F / 14C / 1P / per serving

½ cup popcorn kernels
1 cup white chocolate chips
1 serving CSE Super Berry Mix
Dash sea salt

1. Use an air popper to pop your popcorn into a large bowl. Sift through the popcorn and remove all unpopped kernels.

2. Place the chocolate into a microwave safe bowl and microwave 30 seconds at a time, stirring in between, until chocolate is completely melted and smooth. Usually takes 60-90 seconds total to melt.

3. Stir the Super Berry Mix into the chocolate and then pour over the popcorn. Use a rubber spatula to stir the popcorn until well coated. Pour out onto a cookie sheet or wax paper to let the chocolate set. Sprinkle sea salt over the top to taste. Enjoy!

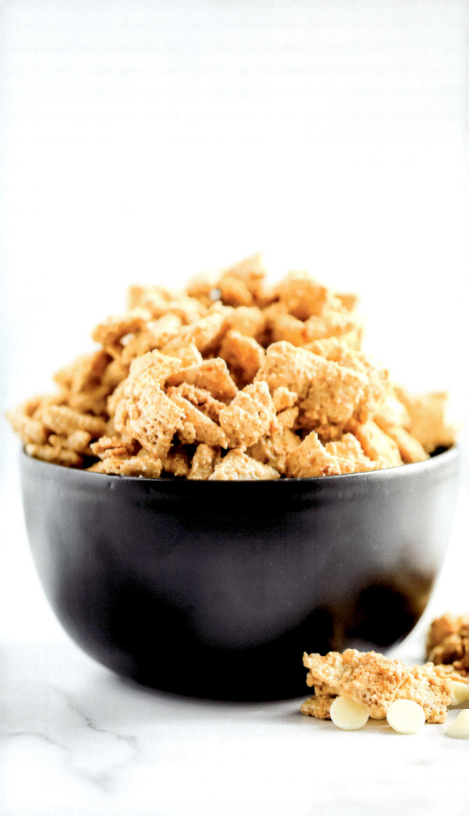

WHITE CHOCOLATE CINNAMON PUPPY CHOW

Makes 16 servings
245 calories / 11F / 29.5C / 6.5P / per serving

8 cups (1 box) Cinnamon Chex Cereal
2 Tbs. grass-fed butter
1 cup white chocolate chips
½ cup OffBeat Sweet Classic PB
  or natural peanut butter
1 serving CSE Simply Vanilla Protein Powder
½ cup powdered peanut butter

1. Pour the cereal into a large bowl.

2. Add the butter, white chocolate chips and peanut butter to a small saucepan. Melt the ingredients down over low/medium heat. Whisk constantly until smooth and pourable.

3. Pour over the cereal and stir until well coated.

4. Dump into a large Ziploc bag and top with the protein powder and the peanut butter powder. Seal the bag and shake until the cereal is well coated. Pour back into the bowl and enjoy! Store extras in the fridge.

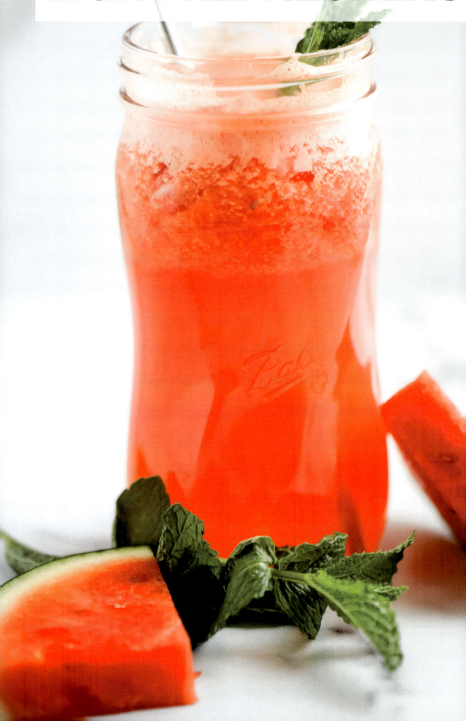

LIGHT REFRESHERS

SIP, SIP HOORAY!

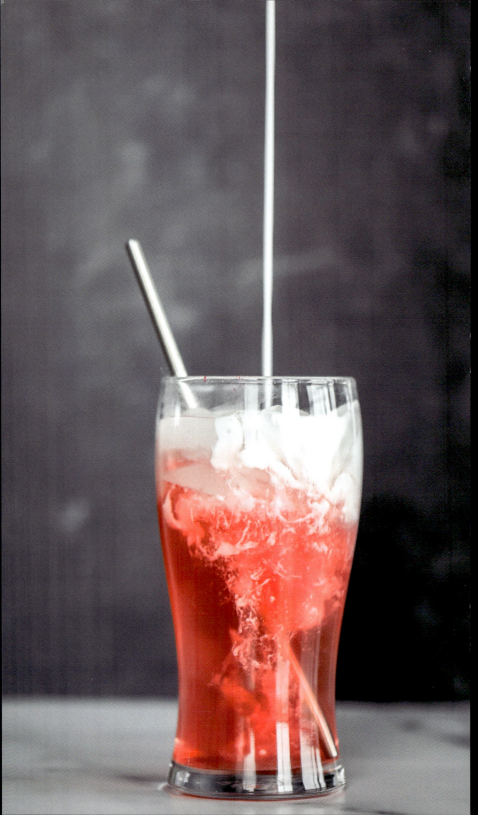

CSE ITALIAN SODA

Makes 1 serving
45 calories / 3F / 4C / 0P

---

1 True Lemon Lemonade single serving packet
8-12 oz. sparkling water, any brand, any flavor
Ice cubes
2 Tbs. lite canned coconut milk
2 Tbs. spray whipped cream

1. Pour the True Lemon Lemonade into a 16 oz. cup, then pour the sparkling water over the top. Add in a handful of ice cubes and stir. Add in the coconut milk and top with whipped cream. Enjoy!

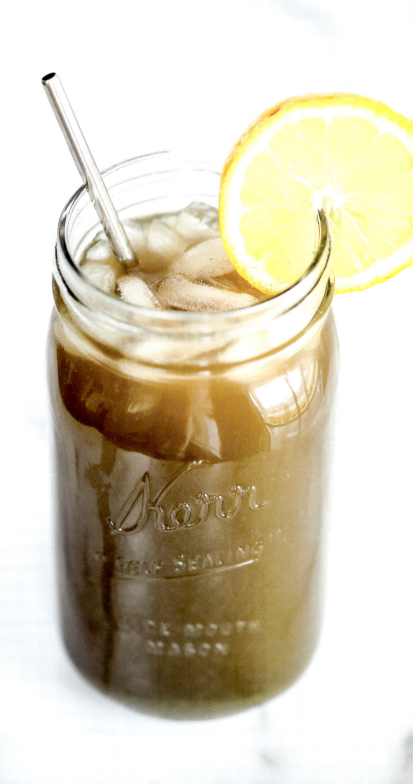

GREEN LEMON TONIC

Makes 1 serving
75 calories / 0F / 21C / 0P

---

16 oz. water
1 serving CSE Super Greens Mix
1 Tbs. apple cider vinegar
1 lemon, juice of
1 Tbs. raw honey
Ice cubes

1. Add all of the ingredients to a large glass. Whisk with a milk frother, a whisk or shake in a shaker cup. Enjoy with a straw!

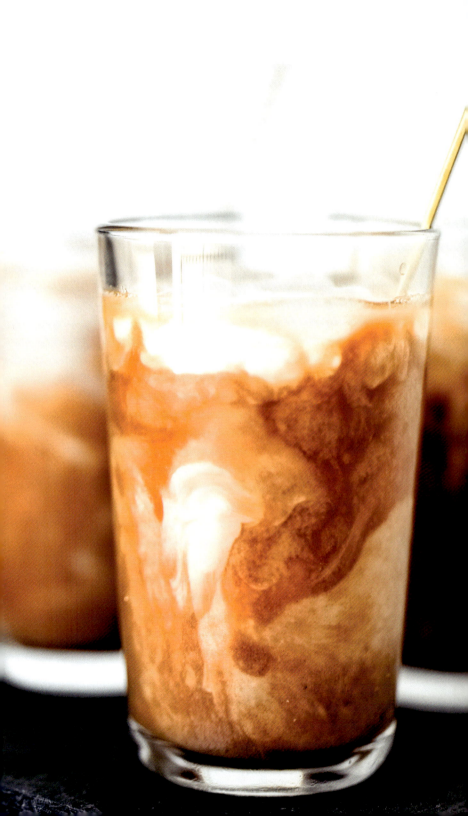

ICED CRIO
Makes 1 serving
80 calories / 4F / 10C / .5P

½ cup Crio Concentrate (recipe below)
½ cup unsweetened almond milk
1 Tbs. full-fat, canned coconut milk
2 tsp. organic coconut sugar
Vanilla stevia drops, to taste
Ice cubes

1. Add all the ingredients to a shaker cup (except the ice) and shake until the sugar is dissolved.

2. Pour into a glass full of ice. Enjoy cold with a straw.

Crio Concentrate
Makes 24 ounces

4 cups water
1 cup Crio Bru grounds, any flavor

1. Add water and Crio Bru to a saucepan and bring to a light boil. Simmer for 10 minutes.

2. Let cool slightly then drain the grounds by either running it through a coffee filter or by using a French press. Pour into an air-tight jar or container and refrigerate.

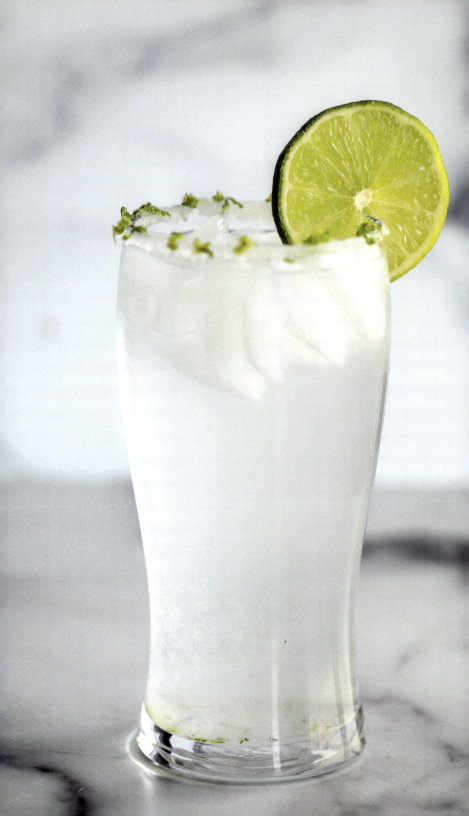

LIME RICKEY

Makes 1 serving
8 calories / 0F / 2C / 0P

16-24 oz. cold water
1 lime, juice of
Vanilla stevia drops, to taste
Ice cubes

1. Add all of the ingredients to a large cup or water bottle. Mix and enjoy!

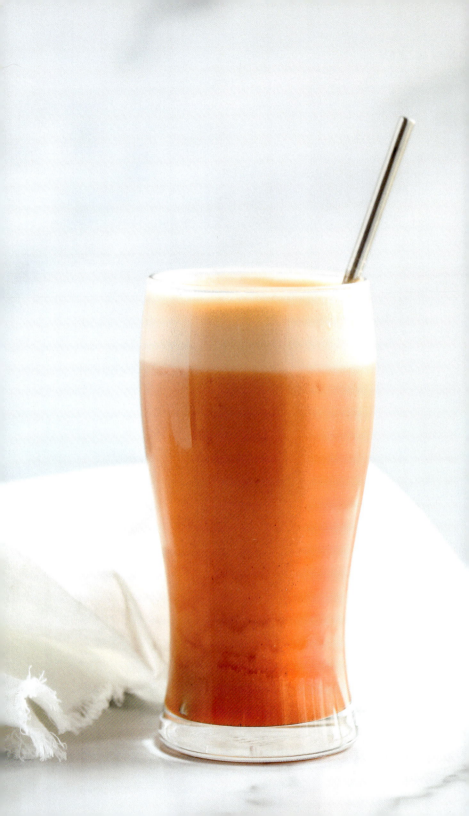

PEACH BERRY ENERGY DRINK

Makes 1 serving
65 calories / 0F / 11C / 5P

8-10 oz. coconut water
1 serving CSE Super Berry Mix
1 serving CSE Peach Mango Super Collagen Mix
8-10 (120g) ice cubes

1. Add all ingredients to a high-powered blender. Blend until smooth.

2. Pour into a cup and enjoy!

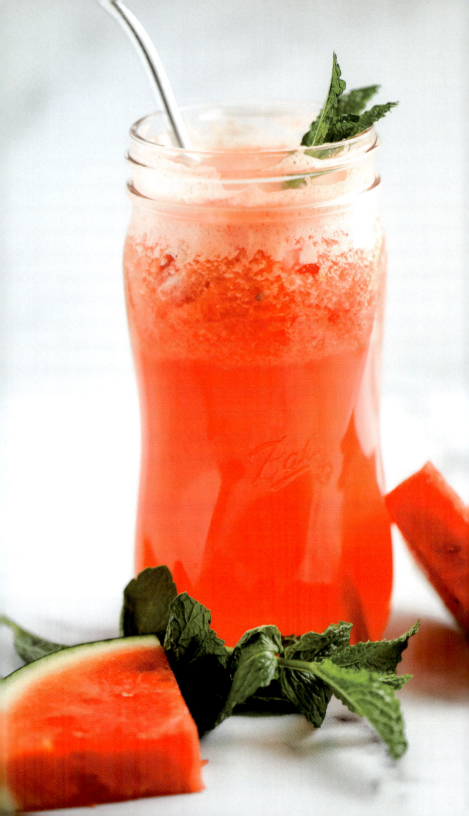

WATERMELON LEMONADE

Makes 1 serving
55 calories / 0F / 14.5C / 1P

---

16 oz. cold water
1 cup fresh watermelon
1 lemon, juice of
Vanilla stevia drops, to taste
Ice cubes
Fresh mint, optional

1. Add the water, watermelon, lemon juice and stevia drops to a blender. Blend on high until smooth.

2. Pour into a glass with ice and fresh mint. Enjoy!

CLEAN

SIMPLE

SWAPS

WHITE, WHOLE-WHEAT FLOUR, WHOLE WHEAT PASTRY FLOUR, KODIAK CAKES MIX	KODIAK CAKES GLUTEN-FREE MIX, BOB'S RED MILL GLUTEN-FREE ALL-PURPOSE BAKING FLOUR, KING ARTHUR GLUTEN-FREE FLOUR OR ALL-PURPOSE MIX OR THRIVE MARKET PALEO FLOUR
GRASS-FED BUTTER	COCONUT OIL
DARK CHOCOLATE CHIPS	ENJOY LIFE CHOCOLATE CHIPS OR NESTLE TOLLHOUSE SIMPLY DELICIOUS SEMI-SWEET MORSELS
WHITE CHOCOLATE CHIPS	KING DAVID WHITE CHOCO CHIPS O ARTISAN KETTLE WHITE CHOCOLATE CHIPS
GREEK YOGURT	PLAIN KITE HILL ALMOND MILK YOGURT, PLAIN FORAGER CASHEW-GURT OR PLAIN SO DELICIOUS COCONUT MILK YOGURT
CREAM CHEESE	TRADER JOE'S, KITE HILL OR MIYOKOS VEGAN CREAM CHEESE STYLE SPREAD
WHIPPED CREAM	ALMOND MILK REDDI WIP OR COCONUT MILK REDDI WIP
XYLITOL	SUGAR IN THE RAW
BUTTERSCOTCH CHIPS	KING DAVID BUTTERSCOTCH CHIPS
BUTTER EXTRACT	VANILLA OR ALMOND EXTRACT
FAT-FREE MILK	CASHEW MILK, COCONUT MILK OR ALMOND MILK
WHEY PROTEIN POWDER	VEGAN PROTEIN POWDER

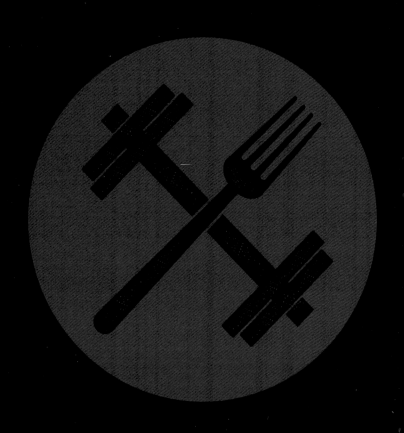

WWW.CLEANSIMPLEEATS.COM